REFLEXES, LEARNING and BEHAVIOR

A Window Into the Child's Mind

by

Sally Goddard

*A NON-INVASIVE APPROACH TO SOLVING
LEARNING & BEHAVIOR PROBLEMS*

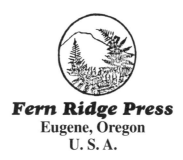

Fern Ridge Press
Eugene, Oregon
U. S. A.

Publisher's Data in Publication

Goddard, Sally, 1957-
Reflexes, learning and behavior, a window into the child's mind.
Eugene, Oregon, Fern Ridge Press. 2002.
200 p. 10 in, il., Index.
1. Child development. 2. Learning disabilities. 3. Reflexes - testing. 4. Developmental
Neurophysiology 5. Behavior disorders in children. 6. Educational psychology.
LC4818   370.15   ISBN 0 - 9615332 - 8 - 5

Printed in the United States of America
by Thomson-Shore, Inc., Dexter, MI 48130
Typeset digitally by
Editing & Design Services, Inc.
Child illustrations by Dan Chen

Fern Ridge Press
1927 McLean Blvd
Eugene, OR 97405
(541) 485-8243 FAX (541) 687-7701
www.fernridgepress.com

Table of Contents

Chapter 1

Chapter 2

Chapter 3

Chapter 4

Chapter 5

Chapter 6

Chapter 7

Appendix

ACKNOWLEDGEMENTS

To Peter Blythe, who started this work in 1969 and established The Institute for Neuro-Physiological Psychology (INPP) in 1975. He has provided inspiration, education and encouragement to students, professionals and colleagues for over 25 years, and given hope to many thousands of children and their parents. The techniques used by INPP have now spread to the other side of the world, and people talk about the impact of reflexes on learning and behavior — sometimes without knowing the source from which their knowledge stems. Many others have gone on to continue to develop techniques in the light of new knowledge and research. The guiding hand remains that of its founder —

"between the idea and the reality is the creator"

Catharina Johannesson Alvegård, who first developed this work in Sweden.

Dr. Kjeld Johansen.

Dr. Lawrence Beuret, Thake Hansen-Lauff, Björn Gustaffson, Håkan Carlsson, Sheila Dobie, Mary O'Connor and Joan Young.

Professor Birger Kaada at the University of Stavanger, whose work on the *Fear Paralysis Response* provided a vital link, and Ernest Keeling who first introduced INPP to the Fear Paralysis Response.

To many, many other people whose work behind the scenes, discussion, argument and ideas have contributed to the development of this book.

To Svea Gold, whose tireless patience in seeking a solution to children's problems, whose own writing, encouragement and support has helped this book to be.

To my children, James, Thomas and Gabriella, who have allowed me to grow up a second time with them.

PREFACE

There is a famous etching by Hogarth: *Columbus Breaking the Egg*. It depicts the scene in which Columbus, just returned from having discovered the "Indies," is surrounded by his jealous friends. The story goes that they mocked his achievement, saying that his discovery was nothing and they also could have done it.

Calmly (it was said) Columbus picked up an egg from a platter on the table, and asked his detractors to stand the egg on its tip. They tried it, each one, and the egg kept rolling on its side. Finally, Columbus picked up the egg, gave it one short sharp crack on the table, and the egg stood up! His friends laughed and said, "Heck!" (Or whatever language they used at the time) "We could have done that too!" "Yes," answered Columbus. "But I did it!"

Now, whether that story is true or only apocryphal, each science, through the years, had men who cracked the Egg of Columbus and ushered in a whole new era in their field. There was Galileo, Einstein, Pasteur, the Wright brothers — the number is endless.

In 1986 Rita Levi-Montalcini won the Nobel Prize for her work with Nerve Growth Factors. She proved that certain chemicals, usually created at the junction between the nerve and the moving muscle, allowed new connections to be made from the nerve cell. Embryonic egg research had been going on since the early 1920s! Then came Jean-Pierre Changeux and he literally created an Egg of Columbus. He had noticed that chick embryos make certain reflexive movements during their gestation period. While they were in the egg, he took a very fine needle and paralyzed their muscles with curare, so that these reflexive movements could not take place. Then, when the chicks emerged, he examined the chicks' brain, and the brains showed abnormalities!

At the time I wrote to him and said that his work would be important to children and child development, and he answered that this was the aim behind all his research, but it would be a long way off.

What Changeux did not know, was that just at the time Peter Blythe together with David McGlown was looking at children who had trouble in school — children who had been labeled "Minimal Brain Damage"— and he found that these children, overwhelmingly, showed signs of retained reflexes, reflexes that should have disappeared long ago. They also seemed to miss postural reflexes that should have been there. This was a neurological profile, quite different from that of children who had no problems. Now developmental therapies have been around for a long time —. since about the fifties, I would say. Children's development, also, has been studied for a long time, ever since the Gesell Institute started to document what milestones of development to expect from the growing child. With this knowledge, reflex therapy was used on cerebral palsied children and stroke patients, but it remained for Peter Blythe and Sally Goddard to use this knowledge to help the "puzzle" children: those children who to all intents and purposes seemed normal. We blamed them for unacceptable behavior or labeled them stupid - because we did not understand them.

At the Institute for Neuro-Physiological Psychology they showed how to look for reflexes, they coded the evaluations so that it became possible to get an accurate insight into what it was that affected a child's behavior. Exactly how did each reflex affect a child? Once a profile of the child's reflexes was discovered to have failed to develop in the expected order, what could be done to help this child? It was not a theoretical, laboratory kind of research: it provided application in ways that parents, teachers and doctors can use.

Already optometrists are using this knowledge to speed up visual training. From Sweden to Australia - wherever Sally Goddard's first book has reached — teachers are using the information to have a new awareness of what makes one child succeed and another fail. In the United States, some teachers provide "wiggle cushions" for children who can't sit still, because they realize these children may have a retained Spinal Galant. Some provide elastic bands tied around the legs of chairs to help children counteract the effects of a retained symmetrical tonic neck reflex. They no longer undermine Johnny's self esteem by telling him: "You're not writing with your tongue!" They know that he still has signs of a Babkin response. With this new approach there is peace and quiet in the classroom and teachers have a chance to teach instead of just wasting time in keeping the class disciplined. After the temporary stopgap methods are used, physical programs are being instituted to have each child reach the milestones needed to succeed. I have used the Institute's techniques in my work with juvenile delinquents and their turn-around has been stunning!

Jean-Pierre Changeux's egg research has become useful sooner than he thought — it backs up the rationale behind Peter Blythe's reflex stimulation/inhibition program. But it took the work of the Institute for Neuro-Physiological Psychology to stand the egg on its head!

Svea Gold
January 2002

INTRODUCTION

Parents are usually the first people to recognize when a child has a problem. Often they do not know what is wrong, they simply sense: "There is something different about my child." Unless the symptoms are severe, the difficulties are often overlooked and parents are told: "He will grow out of it!" What is almost worse is that they themselves are often dismissed as being over-anxious or even neurotic parents.

While it is certainly true that many children do grow out of early problems and there are many individual variations within recognized stages of development, there exist also a group of children who, to all outward appearances are "normal," but who are immature in other aspects of their development. If these immaturities persist, the children are at risk of experiencing a range of learning and behavior difficulties at various stages in their lives.

Research in the area of neural plasticity has shown us that the "wiring" of the central nervous system is open to change, particularly in its stages of most rapid growth or maturation, and that this rewiring has a profound impact upon a child's ability to interact effectively with both their social and physical environment. Galaburda (2001) suggests that problems can arise from two levels in the brain: higher and lower order processing. While it is generally accepted that during the process of maturation, higher centers in the brain should take increasing control and direction over lower centers, the persistence of lower level dominance over certain functions will nevertheless have an effect on how a child functions, its ability to learn and its behavior.

Most education and many remedial techniques are aimed at reaching higher centers in the brain. A Neuro-Developmental approach identifies the lowest level of dysfunction and aims therapy at that area. Once problems there have been remedied, it attempts to build links from lower to higher centers through the use of specific stimulation techniques.

All learning takes place in the brain; it is the body that acts as receptor for information and then becomes the vehicle through which knowledge is expressed. In this respect, movement lies at the heart of learning. Learning, language and behavior are all linked in some way to the function of the motor system and control of movement. Before our children learn to talk, we read their language through gesture, alteration in posture, rhythm of movement, pitch, volume and tone of voice.

Speech as a skill is dependent upon the motor system for the combination of movements involved in coordinating the larynx, the pharynx, the tongue and the muscles at the front of the mouth. Reading depends largely on oculo-motor skill involving precise eye movements and writing involves hand-eye coordination with the support of the postural system. Most academic learning depends on basic skills becoming automatic at the physical level. If a child fails to develop automatic control over balance and motor skills, many other aspects of learning can be affected negatively, even though the child has average or above average intelligence.

Control of the body also lays the foundation for self-control. Immaturity in the functioning of the nervous system is often accompanied by signs of emotional immaturity such as poor impulse control, difficulty in reading the body language of others (social cues) and unsatisfactory peer relationships. One parent described his child as being: "ten years old on the outside and three years old on the inside." No amount of behavior modification made a difference to his son's emotional behavior until the underlying problem of Neuro-Developmental Delay had been addressed.

Making the Child Fit The System...

When children first enter formal school (in the UK at rising 5 years of age), it is generally assumed that they will be able to sit still, pay attention, hold a writing implement and get their eyes to make the movements necessary to follow along a line of print. Many children do acquire these skills without difficulty; others take longer because they enter the school system at a definite disadvantage in terms of their neurological development and therefore lack the necessary physical abilities to succeed. In the higher grades these children run the risk of experiencing what is labelled specific learning difficulties, not because they lack intelligence, but because the basic systems fundamental to learning were not fully in place at the time they started school. Attention, Balance and Coordination are the primary A, B and C upon which all later academic learning depends.

The concept of maturational readiness for learning is not new. As early as 1947, it was noted that reading readiness seemed to coincide with the shedding of the first milk teeth, and that individual variation in the timing of the eruption of the second tooth might be indicative of other aspects of neurological maturity related to reading readiness (Ames 1967). In 1999, Bax and Whitmore investigated whether it would be of value to include a short test battery of neuro-developmental tests in school entrant medical examinations. They found that there were significant links between neurological maturity and performance on cognitive psychological tests. Despite an increasing body of evidence to support the value of neuro-developmental milestones at the time of school entry, these tests have still not been integrated into standard school pre-assessment. Chronological age alone still remains the criterion on which we allow a child to enter school.

Such a blanket approach to starting a child's formal education can adversely affect at least two groups: Those children whose birthdays fall in the summer and who are therefore 9-12 months younger than their peers, and those children who are delayed in certain aspects of development related to the automatic control of balance and coordination and who therefore lack the ability to focus and sustain attention. The former can benefit simply by delaying time of school entry by several months and thus allowing the child to enter as one of the older children in the next year's group. Those who had not yet achieved certain developmental milestones would benefit from an extended period of a more informal curriculum that included increased activities to foster physical and sensory development.

In the former Czechoslovakia two simple tests were used to assess school readiness: Could the child draw a circle in both a clockwise and anti-clockwise direction? (This basic movement is involved in forming letters when writing.) Could the child touch one ear with the opposite hand and repeat this on the other side? (This shows whether a child is able to cross the midline of the body — a skill needed for the act of reading.)

Independent research has found similar connections between control of automatic balance and later learning abilities, and a number of tests such as "The Wobble Test (Nicolson and Fawcett 1994) and the One Leg Stand (Schrager 2001) have been incorporated into more extensive test batteries to identify children who have, or who are at risk of having dyslexia and other specific learning disabilities. While these tests provide indications of what is wrong, they do not tell us why one child has gained a degree of control over balance and coordination and another child has not.

It is the purpose of this book to provide not only the **WHY**, but to suggest the **HOW** to identify the child at risk and overcome the obstacles which keep children from succeeding in school and in life.

Chapter 1

REFLEXES –
Their Impact on Success
or Failure in Education

When a child is born, he leaves the cushioning and protection of the womb to enter a world where he is assailed by an almost overwhelming amount of sensory stimuli. He cannot interpret the sensations that envelop him. If they are too strong, or too sudden, he will react to them, but he does not understand his own reaction. He has exchanged a world of equilibrium for one of chaos; he has left warmth for heat and cold. Automatic sustenance is no longer available and he must start to participate in feeding himself. No longer furnished with oxygen from the mother's blood, he needs to breathe for himself, and he must start to seek and to find the fulfillment of his own needs.

To survive, he is equipped with a set of primitive reflexes designed to insure immediate response to this new environment and to his changing needs. Primitive reflexes are automatic, stereotyped movements, directed from the brain stem and executed without cortical involvement.

Conscious awareness is possible only when the cortex becomes involved in the event.

They are essential for the baby's survival in the first few weeks of life, and they provide rudimentary training for many later voluntary skills. The primitive reflexes, however, should only have a limited life-span and, having helped the baby to survive the first hazardous months of life, they should be inhibited or controlled by higher centers of the brain. This allows more sophisticated neural structures to develop, which then allow the infant control of voluntary response.

If these primitive reflexes remain active beyond 6-12 months of life, they are said to be aberrant, and they are evidence of a structural weakness or immaturity within the central nervous system (CNS). Prolonged primitive reflex activity may also prevent the development of the succeeding postural reflexes, which should emerge to enable the maturing child to interact effectively with his environment. Primitive reflexes retained beyond six months of age may result in immature patterns of behavior or may cause immature systems to remain prevalent, despite the acquisition of later skills. One parent described his child as "having an infant still active within a ten-year-old's body."

Depending on the degree of aberrant reflex activity, this poor organization of nerve fibers can affect one or all areas of functioning: not only gross muscle and fine muscle co-ordination, but also sensory perception, cognition and avenues of expression. The fundamental equipment essential for learning will be faulty or inefficient despite adequate intellectual ability. It is as if later skills remain tethered to an earlier stage of development and instead of becoming automatic, can only be mastered through continuous conscious effort.

The primitive reflexes emerge in utero, are present at birth, and should be inhibited by six months of age —twelve months at the latest.

Inhibition of a reflex frequently correlates with the acquisition of a new skill. Thus knowledge of reflex chronology and normal child development may be combined to predict which later skill may have been impaired as a direct result of retained primitive reflexes. In much the same way that the parent used the analogy of an infant remaining active in a schoolboy's body, it may be said that the individual's aberrant reflexes can give us clues as to what is actively hindering later skills.

Detection of primitive reflexes can help to isolate the causes of a child's problem so that remedial training can be targeted more effectively. If the reflex profile is only marginally abnormal, teaching strategies *alone* will usually be sufficient. Children with a moderate degree of reflex abnormality may benefit from a combination of specialized teaching and some motor training designed to improve balance and coordination. If, however, a **cluster** of aberrant reflexes are present, ***neuro-developmental delay*** is said to exist. In such cases, the child will only be able to sustain long term improvement after following a ***reflex stimulation/inhibition program*** designed specifically for him to treat the aberrant reflexes still present.

Perception is the registering of sensory information in the brain.

Cognition is the interpretation and understanding of that information.

Inhibition - suppression of one function through the development of another. The first function becomes integrated within the second.

Disinhibition occurs after trauma or in Alzheimer's disease when reflexes re-emerge in their reverse chronological order.

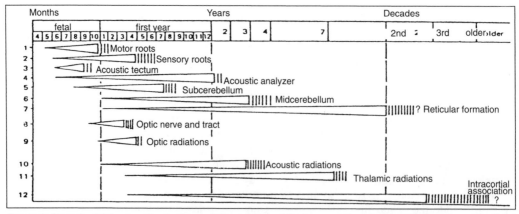

Figure 1: Periods of Intensive Myelination in Different Neural Systems — From before birth to beyond the third decade of life. — *from The Brain by Mildred Robeck*

A *reflex stimulation/inhibition program* consists of specific physical, stereotyped movements practiced for approximately five to ten minutes per day over a period of nine to twelve months. The movements involved are based upon a detailed knowledge of reflex chronology and normal child development. Thelan (1979) observed that all human babies make a series of stereotyped movements during their first year of life. The Institute for Neuro-Physiological Psychology in the United Kingdom and Sweden, maintain that specific movement patterns made in the first months of life contain within them a natural inhibitor to the reflexes, and that if a child has never made these movements in the correct sequence, the primitive reflexes may have remained active as a result. By the application of stylized sequential movements, practiced daily, it is thus possible to give the brain a "second chance" to register the reflex inhibitory movement patterns which should have been made at the appropriate stage in development. As aberrant reflex activity is corrected, many of the physical, academic and emotional problems of the child will disappear.

*Reflex —
an involuntary response
to a stimulus and the
entire physiological
process activating it.*

Each reflex has a vital part to play in setting the stage for later functioning. In order to understand what goes wrong when reflexes become aberrant, it is important to realize what job individual reflexes perform at the time that their presence is normal. To do this, we need to return to the earliest weeks of an embryo's life — just five weeks after conception.

At this time the embryo starts to show signs of response to external stimuli. Gentle touch to the upper lip will cause the embryo to **withdraw** immediately from the stimulus — in an amebic-like response. Only a few days later, this area of sensitivity will be spread to include the palms of the hands and the soles of the feet, until eventually the whole body surface is responsive to touch. At this stage, however, the response is always one of **withdrawal** from the source of contact, and is a total body reaction. As tactile awareness develops, withdrawal upon contact gradually lessens.

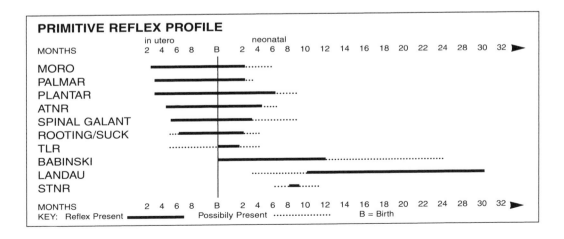

3

It is when the withdrawal reflexes are gradually lessening, estimated at 9 weeks in utero, that the first of the primitive reflexes emerge. The Moro reflex appears at 9-12 weeks after conception and continues to develop throughout pregnancy so that it is fully present at birth.

Neural development —not chronological age— determines at what time each reflex emerges and at what time it becomes inhibited. Thus the presence or absence of reflexes at key stages in development may be used as diagnostic signposts of central nervous system (CNS) maturity.

MORO REFLEX

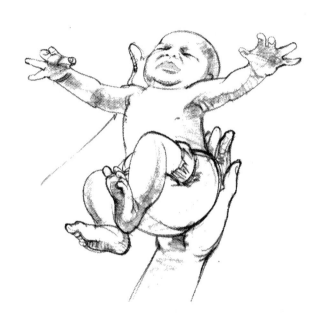

Emerges: 9 weeks in utero
Birth: fully present
Inhibited: 2-4 months of life

TRIGGERS TO THE MORO REFLEX:

1.   Sudden, unexpected occurrence of any kind
2.   Stimulation of the labyrinth by change in head position (Vestibular)
3.   Noise (Auditory)
4.   Sudden movement or change of light in the visual field (Visual)
5.   Pain, temperature change, or being handled too roughly (Tactile)

PHYSICAL RESPONSE TO THE MORO REFLEX.

1.   Instantaneous arousal
2.   Rapid inhalation, momentary "freeze" or "startle" followed by expiration—often accompanied by a cry

3. Activation of "fight or flight" response, which automatically alerts the sympathetic nervous system and results in :
   A. release of adrenaline and cortisol into the system (The stress hormones)
   B. increase in the rate of breathing, particularly in the apices (upper lobes) of the lungs (Hyperventilation)
   C. increase in heart rate
   D. rise in blood pressure
   E. reddening of the skin
4. Possible outburst, e.g. anger or tears

LONG TERM RESPONSE

Poorly developed CO² reflex

The CO² reflex causes spontaneous inhalation of the upper and lower part of the lungs. When CO² levels become too high in the blood, chemical changes take place in the medulla, which will then open the arteries to increase blood supply to the brain and at the same time stimulate deep breathing.

The Moro reflex is a composite series of rapid movements made in response to sudden stimuli. It consists of a sudden symmetrical movement of the arms upward—away from the body—with opening of the hands, momentary freeze and then a gradual return of the arms across the body into a clasping posture. Abduction is accompanied by a sudden intake of breath. Adduction facilitates the release of that breath. Moro in 1918 emphasized his belief that it is essentially a "grasping" reflex, analogous to the one seen in young apes who instinctively cling to their mothers. He called it "Umklammerungsreflex" which literally translated means clasping reflex.

Abduction: opening of the arms and legs outward

Adduction: closing of the arms and legs as if to embrace or to clasp

The Moro reflex is an involuntary reaction to threat. The baby cannot yet analyze incoming sensation to assess whether that threat is real or not. The brain stem releases an immediate Moro response as if an emergency trip-switch were triggered automatically. It acts as the earliest form of "fight or flight" response and may be triggered occasionally in later life in situations of extreme danger. Essentially, however, it should be inhibited in its crude form from 2 to 4 months of age to be replaced by an adult startle reflex or Strauss reflex.

Its role as a survival mechanism in the first months of life is to alert, to arouse and to summon assistance. It is also thought to play a major part in developing the baby's breathing mechanism in utero, coinciding with the earliest breathing-like movements observed in the womb. It facilitates the first "breath of life" at birth and helps to open the windpipe if there is threat of suffocation.

If the Moro reflex fails to be inhibited at 2-4 months of life, the child will retain an exaggerated startle reaction which may result in continued hypersensitivity in one or several sensory channels, causing him to over-react to certain stimuli. Sudden noise, light, movement or alteration of position or balance—any of these—may elicit the reflex at unexpected moments, so that the child is constantly "on alert" and in a heightened state of awareness. The Moro-directed child is poised on the edge of fight or flight through most of his waking moments, caught up in a vicious circle in which reflex activity stimulates the production of adrenaline and cortisol—the stress hormones. These same hormones increase sensitivity and reactivity so that both the trigger and the response are built into the system. Such a child may present a paradox—acutely sensitive, perceptive and imaginative on the one hand, but immature and over-reactive on the other. He may cope in one of two ways: by being the fearful child who "withdraws" from situations, has difficulty in socializing, and can neither accept nor demonstrate affection easily. On the other hand, he may become the over-active, aggressive child, who is highly excitable, cannot read body language and who needs to dominate situations. Either child will tend to be manipulative, as he attempts to find strategies which will give him some measure of control over his own emotional responses.

Adrenaline and cortisol are two of the body's chief defenses against allergy and infection. If they are in constant use as "Leitmotif" in the child's life, they are diverted from their primary function, and there may be insufficient stores available to provide good immunity and balanced response to potential allergens. This may be the child who picks up every cough and cold in circulation and who over-reacts to certain medication. The child may be sensitive to certain foods or food additives, which in turn will affect behavior and concentration. He will also tend to burn up blood sugar quicker than other children, which will further exacerbate swings in mood and performance.

The child who still has a Moro reflex will experience the world as too full of bright, loud and abrasive sensory stimuli. The eyes will be drawn towards changes in light and to every movement within his visual field. His ears may receive too much auditory information. He cannot filter out or occlude extraneous stimuli, so he becomes easily overloaded. He is, in effect, "stimulus bound."

As Arnheim (1969) said, "Too many impressions which arrive from several sensory sources and which fall simultaneously on a mind which has not yet experienced them separately, will fuse for that mind into a single undivided object."

What then are the symptoms which a parent or a teacher might recognize as being suggestive of a strongly residual or retained Moro reflex?

LONG TERM EFFECTS OF RETAINED MORO REFLEX.

1. **Vestibular related problems such a motion sickness, poor balance and coordination, particularly seen during ball games**

In the first 2-4 months of life, at the time when the Moro reflex is active, an infant's visual attention is drawn to the outside edges of shape and form and to sudden movement or change of light on the periphery of vision. If this continues, the child has difficulty ignoring peripheral visual stimuli and maintaining visual attention on the center. This can contribute to distractibility in the older child.

2. **Physical timidity**
3. **Oculomotor and visual-perceptual problems, e.g. stimulus bound effect (cannot ignore irrelevant visual material within a given visual field, so the eyes tend to be drawn to the perimeter of a shape, much to the detriment of perception of internal features)**
4. **Poor pupillary reaction to light, photosensitivity, difficulty with black print on white paper. The child tires easily under fluorescent lighting**

In bright light the pupils should automatically contract to reduce the amount of light entering the eye. In dim light, they should rapidly dilate to allow maximum light to reach the retina. Failure to do this may result in photosensitivity and/or poor night vision.

5. **Possible auditory confusion resulting from hypersensitivity to specific sounds. The child may have poor auditory discrimination skills, and have difficulty shutting out background noise.**
6. **Allergies and lowered immunity, e.g. asthma, eczema, or a history of frequent ear nose and throat infections**
7. **Adverse reactions to drugs**
8. **Poor stamina**
9. **Dislike of change or surprise—poor adaptability**
10. **Poorly developed CO_2 reflex**
11. **Reactive hypoglycemia**

*** *While other residual reflexes tend to have an impact on specific skills, it is the Moro which has an overall effect on the emotional profile of the child.* ***

POSSIBLE SECONDARY PSYCHOLOGICAL SYMPTOMS.

1. **Free floating anxiety—"Angst" (continuous anxiety seemingly unrelated to reality)**
2. **Excessive reaction to stimuli**
   A. **Mood swings—labile emotions**
   B. **Tense muscle tone (body armoring)**
   C. **Difficulty accepting criticism, as this child finds it so difficult to change**
3. **Cycle of hyperactivity followed by excessive fatigue**
4. **Difficulty making decisions**
5. **Weak ego, low self esteem**
   A. **Insecurity/Dependency**
   B. **Need to "control" or "manipulate" events**

The adult startle response consists of a shrugging movement, followed by a turn of the head to check for the source of the disturbance, and once that has been identified, the infant proceeds with whatever it was doing.

The Moro reflex is the only one of the primitive reflexes to be connected in some way to each one of the senses. As the earliest primitive reflex to emerge, it forms a corner-stone in the foundation for life and for living. It is essential for the neonate's survival, but its effects are profound if it fails to be inhibited at the correct time and transformed into an *adult startle response.*

PALMAR REFLEX

(The infant grasp reflex)
Emerges: 11 weeks in utero
Birth: Fully present
Inhibited: 2—3 months of life

Transformed: Gradual development from involuntary grasp to release and refined finger control. Replaced by the pincer grip at 36 weeks of age.

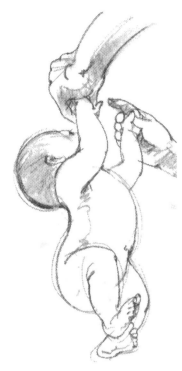

The palmar reflex forms a part of the group of reflexes which develop in utero, and whose common characteristic is to "grasp." A light touch or pressure to the palm of the hand will result in closure of the fingers. By 18 weeks after conception the response will have extended to included a gripping reflex in response to a pull against the finger tendons. Both of these responses should strengthen during uterine life, to be fully developed at birth. They should be strongly active for the first 12 weeks of life and transformed by 4-6 months of life, so that the child can hold an object between his thumb and index finger in a pincer grasp grip. The ability to release an object follows some weeks later and must be practiced many times before the child can acquire good manual dexterity.

Both the palmar and the plantar reflexes are thought to be a continuation of an earlier stage in human evolution, when it was still necessary for the neonate to cling to its mother for safety. There is also a direct link between the palmar reflex and feeding in the early months of life. The palmar reflex can be elicited by sucking movements, and the action of sucking may cause kneading of the hands in time to sucking movements. (Babkin response) Both the mouth and the hands are the major sources of exploration and expression during the neonate period. Continued reflex activity in the area can have a lasting adverse effect upon fine muscle coordination, speech and articulation if they fail to be inhibited at the correct time.

The effects of this neurological loop which connects the palms with the movements of the mouth can often be seen when the child first learns to write or to draw. Until these skills come easily, the child will lick his lips, or twist his mouth some other way. Teachers will often admonish: "You're not writing with your tongue!" Developmental optometrists call this "overflow" and consider the child to have made visual progress when this overflow disappears.

If the palmar reflex remains, the child cannot proceed through the subsequent stages of release and finger mobility. Gesell (1939) described the process as follows: *"Voluntary grasping, such as reaching, indicates a proximo-distal course of development. Early grasping consists of crude palming movements in which the three ulnar fingers predominate, whereas the thumb is practically inactive. This type of grasp is later succeeded by a refined fingertip prehension, characterized principally by thumb opposition, forefinger dominance, readiness for manipulation and the adaption of finger pressure to the weight of the object."* This can only occur as the palmar reflex becomes inhibited.

LONG TERM EFFECTS OF A RETAINED PALMAR REFLEX.

1. **Poor manual dexterity. The palmar reflex will prevent independent thumb and finger movements**
2. **Lack of "pincer" grip, which will affect pencil grip when writing**
3. **Speech difficulties— continuing relationship between hand and mouth movement via the Babkin response will prevent the development of independent muscle control at the front of the mouth, which will then affect articulation**
4. **Palm of the hand may remain hypersensitive to tactile stimulation**
5 . **Child makes movements with mouth when trying to write or draw**

A retained or residual palmar reflex beyond 4-5 months of life will impede both manual dexterity and manipulatory activities. Handwriting will be affected as the child will be unable to form a mature pencil grip. Speech may also be affected as a continuing relationship between hand and mouth movements will prevent the development of independent muscle control at the front of the mouth. Clear articulation may be just one casualty.

Incidentally, André-Thomas and his co-workers (1954) found that it is possible to inhibit the Moro reflex by stimulating the Palmar reflex. When the Moro reflex is activated by shaking the head, the arms, hands and fingers extend. If the Palmar reflex is stimulated first, by placing an object in the palm of one of the hands, the Moro response only occurs in the arm on the side of the open hand. If an object is placed in both hands, the Moro reaction seems to be inhibited in the arms bilaterally. Subconsciously, we sometimes utilize this effect. When about to undertake an unpleasant or difficult task, or in anticipation of a temporarily painful stimulus such as an injection, we often clasp and unclasp our hands. Stress balls may be effective as a result of the same principle. The observations indicate that early reflexes can operate in two ways: either in a chain reaction, or with one reflex having an inhibitory affect upon another. It is these principles which underlie the programs upon which reflex stimulation and inhibition remedial techniques are based.

Proximo-distal: development of the infant's muscle control from the center outward.

Ulnar: first three fingers.

ASYMMETRICAL TONIC NECK REFLEX

Emerges:
18 weeks in utero
Birth: Fully present
Inhibited:
About 6 months of life

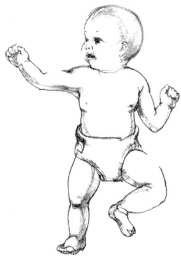

Movement of the baby's head to one side will elicit reflexive extension of the arm and leg to the side to which the head is turned and flexion of the occipital limbs.

The asymmetrical tonic neck reflex (ATNR) has an active part to play from the time of its emergence in utero, until approximately six months of life. During uterine life, the asymmetrical tonic neck reflex should facilitate movement (the kick), develop muscle tone and provide vestibular stimulation.

The ATNR in utero provides continuous motion which stimulates the balance mechanism and increases neural connections.

It should be fully established by the time the fetus is ready to be born, so that it may participate in the birth process. Labor should not begin until the fetus has reached maturity when the fetus releases a hormone into the mother's bloodstream which stimulates contractions of the uterus. Mother and baby may then act as cooperative partners in the birth process. As the second stage of labor is achieved, the baby should help to "unscrew" itself down the birth canal in rhythm with the mother's contractions. It is thought that the ATNR together with the neck righting reflex of the body and Spinal Galant reflex lend flexibility and motility to the shoulders and hips which should assist in the process. The baby's active participation in this is dependent upon the presence of a full asymmetrical tonic neck reflex. The birth process in return reinforces the asymmetrical tonic neck reflex (and other reflexes) so that they are firmly established and active during the first months of life.

Occipital limbs—
arm and leg on the
side to which the
back of the head
is turned.

The ATNR not only assists the birth process but is reinforced by it. This may be one reason why some children who require high forceps delivery or who are taken by Cesarean section are at higher risk for developmental delay.

During the neonate period, the turning of the head to one side, which occurs when the asymmetrical tonic neck reflex is activated, should ensure a free passage of air when the baby is in the prone position. The ATNR helps to increase extensor muscle tone, trains one side of the body at a time, and provides the basis for later reaching movements.

Prone—
lying on the tummy

Extensor—
stretching away
from body

It is more than likely that certain reflexes are crucial for survival in the first months of life and that under-developed Moro and Asymmetrical Tonic Neck reflexes may be a factor in Sudden Infant Death Syndrome (SIDS) — the Moro reflex because it should provide an instant arousal mechanism and the ATNR because it should prevent the baby from lying face down when placed on its tummy. (Goddard 1989, 90, 91)

DeMyer (1980) describes the asymmetrical tonic neck reflex (ATNR) as *"the first eye-hand coordination to take place."* "It is present at the time that visual fixation upon nearby objects is developing, and it seems that the nervous system is making sure that the appropriate arm stretches out towards visualized objects. As the hand touches the object, the seeds of awareness of distance (at arm's length) and eye-hand coordination are sown." (Holt 1991)

By six months of age, the asymmetrical tonic neck reflex (ATNR) should have completed its task and the developing brain should release further movement patterns which contain the inhibitor to the asymmetrical tonic neck reflex, allowing more complex skills to be acquired. Continued presence of an asymmetrical tonic neck reflex (ATNR) will interfere with numerous functions. For example, it is impossible to crawl on the stomach with a fluent cross-pattern movement if the asymmetrical tonic neck reflex persists. Crawling and creeping are important for the further development of hand-eye coordination and the integration of vestibular information with other senses. Myelination of the central nervous system (CNS) is enhanced during these processes.

The child who still has an asymmetrical tonic neck reflex when he learns to walk may find his balance is insecure. Movement of the head to either side will result in straightening of the limbs on that side, upsetting the center of balance and insisting on homolateral movement.

If the child walks with the left hand swinging forward as the left foot moves forward, and conversely with the right hand moving at the same time as the right foot, the result will be a robot-like walk. This walk alerts other children to the fact that there is something different and makes the child an easy target for teasing. In sports, tasks such as throwing and kicking a ball will thus appear awkward and clumsy.

The retained asymmetrical tonic neck reflex will cause difficulty in crossing the midline from one side of the body to the other, so that the child cannot make the transition from merely grasping to manipulating an object with both hands. The child will also not be able to establish a preferred hand, leg or ear and if there is no dominant side, there will always be a slight hesitancy in the child's movements. Gazzaniga (1973) suggested that unilaterality of brain functioning is important in order to have a central organization point in the brain for processing incoming information. The child who has ambiguity of laterality does not know, for instance, which hand to use to pick up a hammer, a pencil, or a ball. Since this choice does not become automatic, every movement has to be consciously made, and this becomes an unnecessary source of confusion.

The effect of mixed laterality can be failure to send information to the most efficient center in the brain for that skill; competition between two centers may occur which is rather like having two people in the front of a car, both wanting to drive and both trying to navigate.

The 6 month old baby who still has this reflex will find it difficult to make the normal transition from being able to pass an object from one hand to the other. This skill is normally acquired at about 28 weeks. The asymmetrical tonic neck reflex becomes an invisible barrier to crossing the vertical midline. The entire body will still want to execute tasks using one side at a time, and thus fluent interchange of bilateral movement will be impaired.

Eye movements can also be affected as the child will remain "stimulus bound" at the midline. When such a child is asked to follow an object as it is moved slowly in front of him on a horizontal line, there will be a slight hesitancy as the object is moved from one side of his nose to the other. This same hesitancy will also prevent fluency when he later tries to read.

It is only during the second half of the first year that the child starts to acquire good far-distance vision, and a retained asymmetrical tonic neck reflex may tether the child's vision to arm's length, preventing the next stage from proceeding. Tracking or "ocular pursuit" will also be impaired, with later effect upon reading, writing and spelling.

Trying to write and to express ideas at the same time (cognitive process) with an ATNR is rather like being stuck forever on your third or fourth driving lesson; you know the procedures involved, but if you try to do too many things at one time or someone distracts your attention away from the procedures involved, you stall the engine.

For children with a retained ATNR, writing never becomes automatic and therefore they have difficulty with multi-tasking.

In the classroom, handwriting will be the most obvious casualty of a retained asymmetrical tonic neck reflex. Each time the child turns his head to look at the page, his arm will want to extend and the fingers will want to open. Thus, holding and manipulating a writing implement for any length of time, will require enormous effort. The effect is as if an elastic band is attached to the pencil and then tethered to the corner of the table. The child is thus fighting against a perpetual invisible force. He may learn to compensate by using an immature pencil grip or by using excessive pressure, but the physical act of writing will always require intense concentration at the expense of cognitive processing. Both the quality and quantity of handwriting will be affected. Writing may slope in different directions from one side of the page to the other. The child may rotate the page by as much as 90 degrees when writing in an attempt to "accommodate" the effect of the asymmetrical tonic neck reflex. Fluent expression of ideas in written form may show a marked discrepancy from the child's ability to express himself orally.

SYMPTOMS SUGGESTIVE OF A RESIDUAL OR RETAINED ASYMMETRICAL TONIC NECK REFLEX.

1. **Balance may be affected as a result of head movement to either side**
2. **Homolateral, instead of normal cross-pattern movements, e.g. when walking, marching, skipping, etc.**
3. **Difficulty crossing the midline**
4. **Poor ocular "pursuit" movements, especially at the midline**
5. **Mixed laterality. (Child may use left foot, right hand, left ear, or he may use left or right hand interchangeably for the same task.)**
6. **Poor handwriting and poor expression of ideas on paper**
7. **Visual-perceptual difficulties, particularly in symmetrical representation of figures**

12

ROOTING REFLEX

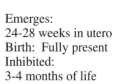

Searching, sucking and swallowing reflexes should be present in all full-term babies. They, also, form part of the group of "grasp" reflexes which develop in utero.

Light touch of the cheek or stimulation of the edge of the mouth will cause the baby to turn the head toward the stimulus, and open the mouth with extended tongue in preparation for sucking. This reflex may be elicited at all four quadrants of the mouth, and thus is sometimes referred to as the cardinal points reflex.

Emerges:
24-28 weeks in utero
Birth: Fully present
Inhibited:
3-4 months of life

The combination of rooting and suck reflexes insure that the baby turns toward the source of food and opens his mouth wide enough to latch on to the breast or bottle. The sucking and swallowing movements which follow are vital for early feeding. Odent (1991) stated that the rooting reflex is at its strongest in the first couple of hours after birth, but if the baby does not receive gratification for his "rooting" attempts shortly after birth, the reflex will weaken. Premature babies who have to be incubated, can frequently be seen "rooting" for the first couple of days of life, but, unable to receive the appropriate response, the rooting reflex starts to diminish. In some of these children, the reflex can still be elicited in weakened form long after it should have been inhibited. In common with other reflexes, if it is not used fully at the correct time, it appears to behave rather like a Victorian spinster—unfulfilled, frustrated and unable to let go!

The strength of the rooting reflex may come and go according to when the last feed was taken. It disappears temporarily after the infant is satiated to reappear only after some time has elapsed. Conversely, it can appear as a "vacuum" activity without the external stimulus of touch in the hungry infant who will turn the head in all directions seeking sustenance.

Peiper (1963) suggests that primitive reflex activity leads an infant into the next stage of a conditioned reflex and he cites the rooting reflex as an example of this. *"When we touch the region of the infant's mouth, reflexes are elicited that turn the head, and move the lips so that the touching object is drawn into the mouth. This life preserving function is innate, but the ability to turn to the nipple or the bottle when it appears in the field of vision is not. This is rapidly learned. From the rooting reflex there develops a conditioned reflex that at the sight of the breast or the bottle turns the head to the correct position in space."*

Retained or residual oral reflexes will result in continued sensitivity and immature responses to touch in the mouth region—particularly in the area of the lip. The infant may experience difficulty when solid foods are introduced, as a persistent suck reflex will prevent the tongue from developing the mature combination of movements necessary for swallowing, and remains too far forward in the mouth to allow effective chewing. Copious dribbling which continues into school age may be one result, as both reflexes prevent the child from gaining adequate control of the muscles at the front of the mouth. Manual dexterity may also be affected as immature sucking and swallowing movements continue to affect the hands, causing involuntary palming movements to occur in time with sucking. (Babkin response)

****

"The stimulus for this reflex consists of deep pressure applied simultaneously to the palms of both hands while the infant is in an appropriate position, ideally supine. The stimulus is followed by flexion or forward bowing of the head, opening of the mouth and closing of the eyes. The reflex can be demonstrated in the newborn, thus showing a hand-mouth neurological link even at this early stage. It fades rapidly, and normally cannot be elicited after 4 months of age. Elicitation of the reflex after this age indicates a cerebral lesion." (Holt 1991)

Supine — lying on the back.

Any further indications of the hand/mouth neurological connection are called Babkin response. Like many other reflexive reactions, the effect can be seen in either direction, in this case from hand to mouth, or mouth to hand.

****

Swallowing, feeding, speech articulation and manual dexterity may all be casualties of residual or retained oral reflexes in the older child. As Roberta Shepherd said, *"The development of normal swallowing and of normal coordination between respiration and oral function are all essential elements in the development of speech. It is thought that the muscular action involved in feeding is an essential preparation for babbling and speech."* (1990)

LONG TERM EFFECTS OF RETAINED ROOTING AND SUCK REFLEXES.

1. **Hypersensitivity around lips and mouth**
2. **Tongue may remain too far forward in the mouth, which will make swallowing and chewing of certain foods difficult—the child may dribble. Lack of mature swallowing movements may cause increased arching of the palate (cathedral palate) and the need for orthodontic treatment later on.**
3. **Speech and articulation problems**
4. **Poor manual dexterity**

SPINAL GALANT

If the baby is held in the ventral or placed in the prone position, stimulation of the back to one side of the spine will result in hip flexion (rotation) to 45 degrees toward the side of the stimulus. It should be present with equal strength bilaterally.

Although Galant eventually gave his name to this reflex, it had been described by Bertolotti in 1904 as a "réflexe dorsolombaire." He observed that stimulation to the skin of the lumbar region resulted in a quick contraction of the dorsal muscles. The response disappeared by two years of age. In 1912 Noica found "une réflexe de la masse musculaire sacrolombaire" to be present in most children but rarely in adults. In 1917 both Veragruth and Galant described similar reactions in normal infants which Veragruth also found to be present in some ill adults.

"When the dorsal skin near and along the vertebral column is stroked, the infant forms an arch with his body; the concavity of the arch is directed toward the stimulated area, and by arching in the opposite direction the infant evades stimulus." (Galant 1917)

Emerges:
20 weeks in utero
Birth: Actively present
Inhibited: 3-9 months of life

Isbert and Peiper (1965) found the response to be more extensive than described by Galant. *"Application of the stimulus results in flexion of the pelvis backward and the ipsilateral leg is extended at the knee and the hip joint is flexed . . . frequently the head position can be changed by stimulation of the anterior surface of the trunk: Stimulation of one side causes turning of the face to the stimulated side."* The last observation seems to provide evidence of the chain reaction that can occur from one reflex to the next, i.e. activation of the spinal Galant reflex sometimes extends into an asymmetrical tonic neck reaction.

Ventral :
Lying on tummy, head and hips not supported.

Ipsilateral:
On the same side.

Lordosis:
Bending of the body forward and inward.

If both sides of the spine are stroked simultaneously from the pelvis to the neck, the Pulgar Marx reflex is elicited. This response involves *"flexion of both legs, lordosis of the spine, elevation of the pelvis, flexion of the arms, lifting of the head, loud crying culminating in apnea and cyanosis, emptying of the bladder, and relaxation and bulging of the rectum with bowel movement; after the reflex has fully developed there is general hypertonia lasting for a few seconds."* (Pulgar Marx 1955). Not all of the features of the reflex are present each time it is activated. The Pulgar Marx reflex should be inhibited by 2-3 months of age. This response is rarely seen in older children with specific learning difficulties. At the Institute for Neuro-Physiological Psychology traces of it have been found in several children who have been given a diagnosis of Asperger's Syndrome and in some children who have a history of continued soiling during the day above age five.

Apnea:
Absence or cessation of breathing.

Cyanosis:
Bluish discoloration of the skin.

Little is known about the functions of the spinal Galant reflex, except that it may take an active role in the birth process. Contractions of the vaginal wall stimulate the lumbar region and cause small rotational movements of the hip on one side, similar to the head and shoulder movements of the asymmetrical tonic neck reflex. In this way, the baby can help to work its way down the birth canal.

It has been suggested (Dickson 1991) that the Galant may act as a primitive conductor of sound in utero, allowing sound vibration to travel up through the body in the aquatic environment of the womb, enabling the fetus to "feel" sound, or assisting sound vibrations to travel up the spinal column. Some weight has been added to this hypothesis by a study carried out by Butler Hall and Hadley which investigated the effect of Auditory Integrative Training (AIT) on abnormal primitive and postural reflexes. AIT is a system of sound therapy developed by Guy Berard for treating a range of listening and language related problems. Butler Hall (1998) found that the spinal Galant reflex was consistently reduced in children as a result of AIT training, suggesting that there is a functional relationship between the spinal Galant reflex and hearing. (see Chapter 4 "The Senses")

Another interpretation offered is that the spinal Galant reflex is a legacy of our evolutionary heritage from the days when we had a tail (Phillips 1994). A tail or tail-like movement is still useful during uterine life for moving in the womb. It might also be useful for balance during the time that a child is creeping and crawling (the quadruped stage of development) and for helping to synchronize upper and lower body movements on one side, but it becomes redundant when the erect posture is achieved when the front of the body and the arms take over some of the adaptive functions of balance and coordination.

If the spinal Galant reflex remains beyond the neonate period, it can be elicited at any time by light pressure in the lumbar region. **Simultaneous** stimulation down both sides of the spine can activate the related Pulgar Marx reflex, which will cause the infant to urinate. A retained or residual spinal Galant reflex is found in many children who may have poor bladder control, and who continue to wet the bed after the age of 5 years. Beuret, (1989) working with adults in Chicago, found the spinal Galant reflex to be present in a high percentage of patients suffering from irritable bowel syndrome.

For the child in the classroom, the most obvious effect of a retained spinal Galant reflex will be difficulty in sitting still for any length of time. This is the "ants in the pants" child who wriggles, squirms and constantly changes body position, as the elastic of the waistband or simply leaning against the back of a chair may activate the errant reflex. Understandably, the child may dislike clothing which is tight around the waist. The reflex may also affect concentration and short-term memory as this constant irritant is always vying for the child's attention.

If the Galant remains present on one side only, it may affect posture, gait and any other form of locomotion. This can result in the illusion of a "limp" or contribute to scoliosis. It may also interfere with the full development of the later amphibian and segmental rolling reflexes, affecting fluency and mobility in physical activities or sports.

Scoliosis :
abnormal curvature
of the spine

SYMPTOMS OF A RETAINED SPINAL GALANT REFLEX

1. **Fidgeting**
2. **Bedwetting**
3. **Poor concentration**
4. **Poor short term memory**
5. **Hip rotation to one side when walking.**

TONIC LABYRINTHINE REFLEX

**TONIC LABYRINTHINE REFLEX
(TLR) FORWARDS**

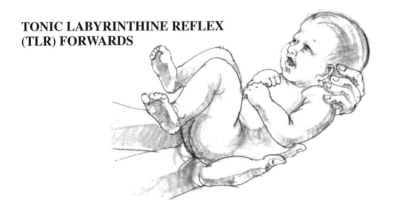

Emerges:
in utero—flexus habitus
Birth: present
Inhibited:
approximately 4 months
of life

TONIC LABYRINTHINE REFLEX (TLR) BACKWARDS.

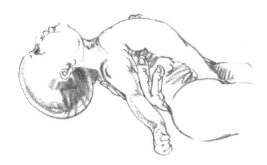

Emerges: at birth
Inhibited: gradual progression from 6 weeks of age up to 3 years of age, involving the simultaneous development of postural reflexes such as the head-righting reflexes and those reflexes usually categorized as postural reflexes but later referred to as "bridging" reflexes such as the symmetrical tonic neck reflex and the Landau reflex.

The Moro and tonic labyrinthine reflexes are closely linked in the early months of life. Both are vestibular in origin, and both are activated by stimulation of the labyrinths, movement of the head and alteration of position in space. The tonic labyrinthine reflex (TLR) is elicited by movement of the head forwards or backwards, above or below the level of the spine. It is thought that flexus habitus (the position of the fetus in utero) is the earliest manifestation of the tonic labyrinthine reflex in the forward position. The tonic labyrinthine reflex in extension is thought to emerge as the baby's head enters the birth canal. The reflex should be fully present from the time of birth. Extension of the head below the level of the spine causes immediate extension of the arms and legs.

The tonic labyrinthine reflex should be fully developed in both positions from birth. Inhibition of the tonic labyrinthine reflex forwards should be accomplished by 4 months of life. Inhibition of the tonic labyrinthine reflex backwards is a more gradual process, involving the emergence of several postural reflexes and taking up to age 3 to be completed.

Being born introduces the baby to an entirely new set of challenges. Hitherto, he has been in an enclosed aqueous environment, in which the effects of all sensory stimuli are cushioned, and the effect of gravity is reduced. The tonic labyrinthine reflex provides him with an early primitive method of response to the problem of gravity. Any movement of the head in a vertical direction beyond the midplane will cause extremes of flexion or extension throughout the body to occur, influencing muscle tone from the head downwards. By 6 months of age the response should be modified as head control develops with the emergence of the oculo- and labyrinthine headrighting reflexes. Head control is an essential prerequisite for the development of all later functions and should be the prime initiator of early movement, tonus and balance. (Cephalo-caudal law)

Cephalo-caudal law: from head to toe downward sequence of development.

The tonic labyrinthine reflexes exerts a tonic influence upon the distribution of muscle tone throughout the body, literally helping the neonate to "straighten out" from the flexed posture of the fetus and the newborn. Thus, balance, muscle tone and proprioception are all trained during this process.

If the tonic labyrinthine reflex fails to be inhibited at the correct time, it will constantly "trip" the vestibular in its actions and in its interaction with other sensory systems. The child who still has a retained tonic labyrinthine reflex when he starts to walk, cannot acquire true gravitational security, (Ayres, 1979-1982) as head movement will alter muscle tone, "throwing" the center of balance. Lacking a secure reference point in space, the child will experience difficulty in judging space, distance, depth and velocity. A sense of direction is based upon our knowledge of where we are in space—if our point of reference is fluctuating and unstable, then the ability to discriminate up from down, left from right and back from front may also be erratic. This is a condition experienced by astronauts in space. When astronauts are put into a gravity free environment, they start to write from right to left, to reverse numbers and letters and to produce "mirror-writing," demonstrating the significance of gravity and balance for orientation, spatial and directional awareness.

Muscle tone: balance between flexor and extensor muscles.

Continued tonic labyrinthine reflex activity will impede the development of the headrighting reflexes. If head control is lacking, eye functioning will also be impaired as the eyes operate from the same circuit in the brain—the vestibulo-ocular reflex arc.

If one segment of the circuit is malfunctioning it will affect the smooth operation of other systems dependent upon that circuit. Balance will be affected by faulty visual information and vision will be affected by poor balance. A two way system of "mismatch" may be established, which the child will assume to be normal because he has never known anything else.

Organization of the vestibular system

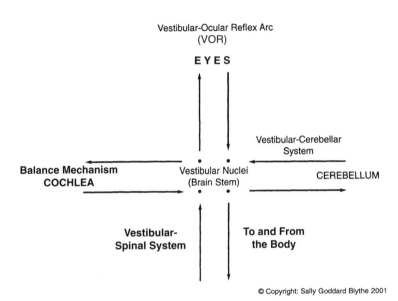

The balance mechanism and the eyes are on the same circuit. Messages from the body pass to the vestibular nuclei and then to the eyes. Messages from the eyes pass to the vestibular nuclei and then to the proprioceptors in the body to make the appropriate adjustments.

© Copyright: Sally Goddard Blythe 2001

A retained Tonic Labyrinthine reflex will affect the messages passing between the vestibular nuclei and the proprioceptors, which in turn will affect the eyes. This will then become a three-way system of mismatch.

The tonic labyrinthine reflex (TLR) may also prevent the child from being able to creep on his hands and knees, as movement of the head will result in extension of the legs. The symmetrical tonic neck reflex (STNR) will also remain "locked" in the system in a futile attempt to over-ride the tonic labyrinthine reflex (TLR) preventing creeping on hands and knees. Crawling and creeping fulfill both training and inhibitory process. Both facilitate integration of sensory information as vestibular, visual and proprioceptive systems all start to operate together for the first time. During that period of developmental movement, the child acquires a sense of balance, a sense of space and a sense of depth. It is through crawling and creeping that the raw materials of seeing, feeling and moving are synchronized for the first time to provide a more complete picture of the environment.

Prolonged influence of the tonic labyrinthine reflex (TLR) can have implications for many other areas of functioning. Balance and movement will be affected. Standing for any length of time may be tiring and posture may have to adjust in an attempt to accommodate the reflex. There may be overall "bowing" of the body or a tendency to stand with the head poked forward. The child may have very floppy muscle tone and appear either slovenly or seem to be jerky and stiff in his movements, particularly in walking, running or jumping. The child may develop a fear of heights as he is intrinsically aware of his poor balance and the fact that movement of his head forwards will cause his knees to bend and create the sensation of falling forwards toward the drop. Holding his arms up will rapidly become tiring, and he will be acutely aware of changes in the level of the ground under his feet, as his feet will attempt to grip the ground as a method of maintaining equilibrium.

Resultant oculomotor dysfunction will cause the eyes to "play tricks" so that he cannot always rely on what he sees. Depth perception may be impaired and he may suffer from figure-ground effect.

****

Figure ground effect: The child cannot easily separate and categorize conflicting visual information. e.g. walking up an open staircase or crossing a slatted bridge, where the water can be seen through the boards. He may have difficulty getting his eyes to readjust from far to near distances, so that there is a temporary "blind spot" in the visual information he receives. Not only will abilities which require spatial perception be affected but he may also have difficulty locating sound and become easily disorientated.

****

Head control and good balance are essential to the automatic functioning of all other systems — a residual tonic labyrinthine reflex (TLR) will prevent the complete establishment of both head control and of balance.

SYMPTOMS SUGGESTIVE OF A STRONGLY RESIDUAL TONIC LABYRINTHINE REFLEX FORWARDS

1. **Poor posture—stoop**
2. **Hypotonus (weak muscle tone)**
3. **Vestibular related problems**
   A. **Poor sense of balance**
   B. **Propensity to get car sick**
4. **Dislike of sporting activities, physical education classes, running, etc.**
5. **Oculomotor dysfunctions**
   A. **Visual-Perceptual difficulties**
   B. **Spatial problems**
6. **Poor sequencing skills**
7. **Poor sense of time**

SYMPTOMS OF A STRONGLY RESIDUAL
TONIC LABYRINTHINE REFLEX BACKWARDS

1. **Poor posture—tendency to walk on toes**
2. **Poor balance and coordination**
3. **Hypertonus—stiff, jerky movements because the extensor muscles exert greater influence than the flexor muscles**
4. **Vestibular related problems**
    A . **Poor sense of balance**
    B.   **Tendency to motion sickness**
5. **Oculomotor dysfunction.**
    A.   **Visual-perceptual difficulties**
    B.   **Spatial perception problems**
6 . **Poor sequencing skills**
7. **Poor organization skills**

SYMMETRICAL TONIC NECK REFLEX

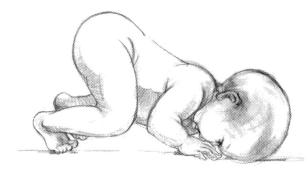

(STNR) **Flexion**.

Emerges:
6-9 months of life.

Inhibited:
9 -11 months of life.

When the child is in the quadruped position, flexion
of the head causes the arms to bend and the legs to extend.

(STNR) **Extension**.

Emerges:
6-9 months of life.

Inhibited:
9 -11 months of life.

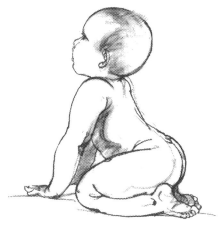

Head extension, on the other hand, causes the legs
to flex and the arms to straighten.

The symmetrical tonic neck reflex has a relatively short life-span. It helps the baby to defy gravity by getting up off the floor on to hands and knees from the prone position. It does not truly belong to either the primitive or the postural reflex categories as it is neither present at birth (primitive reflex) nor should it remain present for life (postural reflex).

Capute (1981) has suggested that it may not be a true reflex, but a crucial stage of the labyrinthine reflex. It certainly helps to inhibit the tonic labyrinthine reflex (TLR) and it forms a bridge to the next stage of locomotion—creeping on hands and knees. However, while it permits the child to assume the quadruped position, it will prevent forward progress in this position. The baby will be at the mercy of its head movement, unable to move effectively because during this period of development the position of the head decides the position of the limbs. (Bobath and Bobath 1955)

Gesell (1947) described progression through the early postural reflexes thus: *"At 20 weeks the supine infant can roll over on his side by rotating the upper portion of the body and then flexing the hips and throwing the legs to that side (segmental rolling reflex). This accomplishment represents the first gross shift in body posture. At 28 weeks, the child can attain a crawling position (full arm extension and amphibian reflex) and sustain the weight of the upper portion of the body by one or both arms. He can bring one knee forward beside the trunk, but cannot raise his abdomen. Locomotion begins at about 32 weeks. The child pivots about by means of his arms. He succeeds in raising himself to the crawling position at 36 weeks (symmetrical tonic neck reflex), but cannot progress on his hands and knees until 44 weeks. It is at this stage that the contralateral arm and leg movements begin."*

Whereas the tonic labyrinthine reflex influences muscle tone throughout the body, the symmetrical tonic reflex effectively divides the body in half at the horizontal midline. When the head is extended, the upper portion of the body also extends and the lower half bends. When the head is flexed, the opposite reaction occurs: the arms bend and the legs straighten. The symmetrical tonic neck reflex seems to "break up" the tonic labyrinthine reflex at the pelvis for a short period of time—just long enough to allow the infant to defy gravity, to adopt the quadruped position and to learn how to use the two halves of the body independently. However, locomotion in both the quadruped and biped positions will require synchrony between the two halves of the body and it is thought that the rocking motion used by many infants just before they learn how to crawl on hands and knees helps to inhibit the symmetrical tonic neck reflex, synchronize functioning of the sacral and occipital areas and enable the child to pass on to the next stage of crawling.

Children who retain the symmetrical tonic neck reflex rarely crawl on hands and knees. They might "bear walk" on their hands and feet, shuffle on their bottoms or simply pull themselves up to standing and walk. Those who do crawl may do so in an unusual fashion: The hands may be rotated outwards to "lock" the elbows and/or the feet may be raised. The crawling pattern will be unsynchronized as the timing of

*Occiput —
back of the head.*

*Sacrum —
derived from the Greek and Egyptian meaning sacred bone, located at the lower end of the spinal column. It consists of five vertebrae fused together to form a triangular bone which lies between the haunch bones and forms the back wall of the pelvis.*

movements in the upper and lower sections of the body do not quite "match."

There can be environmental, developmental and neurological reasons why a child does not crawl. One girl who had been adopted at three years of age had suffered severe environmental deprivation in the first three years of life. She had neither space nor opportunity to crawl. She demonstrated a fully retained symmetrical tonic neck reflex when asked to crawl at seven years of age. Similarly, children who have had little opportunity to play on the floor in the first eight months of life may "bypass" the crawling and creeping stages because they have had insufficient time to develop motor skills in the prone position, which precedes the ability to crawl.

It has been suggested (Blythe 1992) that the symmetrical tonic neck reflex (STNR) helps to complete a sequence of eye training. Bending of the legs as a result of head extension also encourages the infant to "fixate" his eyes at far-distance. Bending of the arms in response to flexion of the head (head lowered below the spine line) will automatically bring the child's focus back to near-distance, thus training the eyes to adjust from far to near distance and back again. The asymmetrical tonic neck reflex (ATNR) begins by extending the baby's ability to focus from about seven inches (17 cm) at birth, to arms length. As the asymmetrical tonic neck reflex (ATNR)is inhibited at about six months of age, the field of vision is extended to distant objects. The symmetrical tonic neck reflex (STNR) then brings the vision back to near-distance once more, training the readjustment of binocular vision. It remains for the process of creeping on hands and knees to further develop the visual skills the infant has learned so far, and to integrate them with information from other senses.

Girls who do not have an STNR, who are put into pretty dresses will sometimes "bear walk" to avoid kneeling on the dress which would otherwise hamper forward movement.

Creeping is one of the most important movement patterns in the prolonged process of teaching the eyes to cross the midline. In addition to looking ahead, babies also learn eye-hand coordination from the movement of the hands. At times, the eyes focus from one hand to another, with the hands acting as moving stimuli. Later on this ability will be essential for being able to read without losing the words at the middle of the line and to visually follow the moving hand when writing. It is through creeping that the vestibular, proprioceptive and visual systems connect to operate together for the first time. Without this integration there can be a poorly developed sense of balance and poor space and depth perception.

The focusing distance and hand-eye coordination skills used in the act of creeping are at the same distance that the child will eventually use for reading and writing. It has been observed (Pavlides 1987) that a high percentage of children with reading difficulties omitted the stages of crawling and creeping in infancy.

Studies of certain primitive tribes have revealed that they possess remarkable visual acuity at far distance, but that they have never developed a written language of their own. The Xinguana Indians can fire a dart from a blow pipe with deadly accuracy as far as half a mile, but they cannot read or write. Within the jungle terrain in which they live, the children spend most of their first year carried upon their mother's body. The ground is fraught with danger from poisonous insects, snakes and plants. Consequently, they are never allowed to learn to crawl or to creep on the ground. Veras (1975) maintains there is a strong connection between crawling and creeping and the ability to comprehend and to use a written language. *"Not only is creeping an important level of development in a child's mobility, it is also terribly important in the child's visual development. In all the primitive people we have seen, the children are never allowed to creep, and none of them can focus his eyes on anything closer than arms length. They are all far sighted. We believe that when a child creeps, his near-point vision is developed."*

Rosanne Kermoian and her colleagues conducted a study at Reed College in 1988 and found that many cognitive skills, such as object permanence and space perception, are learned during the creeping period—and not until then.

Vertical tracking is necessary to align columns correctly when carrying out arithmetical calculations.

Bein-Wierzbinski (2001), using an infra-red computerized eye tracking machine, found the STNR to be a factor in a group of children tested for aberrant eye movements. She found that whereas other reflexes were associated with difficulty with horizontal tracking, the STNR was linked to problems with vertical tracking. When put on to a reflex stimulation/inhibition program the eye movements improved markedly as the reflexes matured.

In the older child, the influence of the symmetrical tonic neck reflex may be seen in a stooped posture, severe slouching, or gradual bending of the arms when sitting at a desk, as head flexion (lowering his head) will cause the arms to bend or collapse. This is the child who ends the lesson almost lying on the desk in order to write.

The child with a symmetrical tonic neck reflex may be the clumsy child who has difficulty coordinating hand and eye movements, dreads physical education classes and is a disaster at ball games. He may lose sight of the ball in motion and by the time he has perceived it at near distance again, it is too late to hit or to catch with any degree of accuracy. Basic skills such as eating may be messy, as the hand never quite seems to be in the right place to find the mouth. Posture at the table, also, will be poor.

In a study carried out by Miriam Bender (1976), a retained STNR was found to be present in 75% of a group of learning disabled children who were compared to a similar group with no learning disabilities. At the Bender Institute, O'Dell and Cook (1996) found a retained STNR to be a significant factor in children with Attention Deficit Disorder (ADD) and Attention Deficit Hyperactive Disorder (ADHD). Both groups improved markedly when the STNR was inhibited as a result of a specific movement program.

SYMPTOMS SUGGESTIVE OF A STRONGLY RESIDUAL SYMMETRICAL TONIC NECK REFLEX.

1. Poor posture
2. Tendency to "slump" when sitting, particularly at a desk or table
3. Simian (ape like) walk
4. "W" leg position when sitting on the floor
5. Poor hand-eye coordination
    A. Messy eater
    B. "Clumsy child" syndrome
6. Difficulties with readjustment of binocular vision (Child cannot change focus easily from blackboard to desk)
7. Slowness at copying tasks
8. Difficulty learning to swim, or unsynchronized movements when swimming above the water. (Often children with a retained STNR swim better under the water where the effect of gravity is reduced and the weight of the water keeps the body level)
9. Can affect attention as a result of discomfort sitting in one position

Chapter 2

FROM PRIMITIVE REFLEX TO POSTURAL CONTROL

If it is the primitive reflexes which lay the foundations for all later functioning, then it is the postural reflexes which form the framework within which other systems can operate effectively. The transition from primitive reflex reaction to postural control is *not an automatic one.* There are no set times at which the later reflex asserts control over the earlier one, but it is a gradual process of interplay and integration during which both reflexes operate together for a short period of time.

As certain movement sequences are practiced over and over again, more mature patterns of response can supersede primitive reflexive response. (Note 1)

The movements made because of the reflex action myelinize brain circuitry in much the same way that the road network of a country is laid out.

This period of growth, change and elaboration operates rather like an interweaving spiral, through which nature ensures that primitive survival patterns are still accessible until such time as more mature postural reactions are becoming automatic.

THE POSTURAL REFLEXES

Postural reflexes are mediated from the level of the midbrain, and their appearance thus signifies the active involvement of higher brain structures over brainstem activity, and are a sign of increased maturity in the central nervous system (CNS). Some posturals are educationally significant.

They comprise two groups:
1.   The Righting Reflexes (Quadruped)
2.   Equilibrium Reactions (Bipedal)
      (Fiorentino 1981).

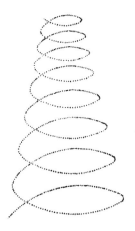

Both are concerned with posture, movement and stability. The righting reactions emerge at 3-12 months of age, and should remain present throughout life until disease or old age intervene. They enable the child to maintain his head and trunk in a specific position when the body position is altered in any way. Their emergence facilitates movement through rolling, crawling and creeping, and later will permit coordinated gross motor movement to take place.

Righting reactions consist of the oculo-headrighting reflex, the labyrinthine headrighting reflex, the amphibian reflex, Landau reflex and segmental rolling reflexes.

Equilibrium reactions do not appear until connections to the cortex are more firmly established. They first appear at approximately 3-6 months of age and persist throughout adult life.

They comprise the protection and tilting reactions which are elicited if balance is lost or the center of gravity altered. They include the *"startle"* (also known as Strauss) reflex and the *parachute* reflex.

> *Educationally, their presence is not of immediate significance, except that* **absence** *of equilibrium reactions suggest immaturity of the Central Nervous System. Socially, however, the impact may be enormous. Because the child will appear clumsy and uncoordinated, he will invite teasing and may become isolated from the group. Organizational skill will also suffer, because balance will be affected, and the resultant dizziness interferes with concentration.* [(Note 2)]

STARTLE PATTERN

The Strauss reflex develops as the Moro reflex is inhibited and it acts as the adult startle response. The child tenses the muscles, blinks, seeks out the source of danger and then makes a cortical (conscious) decision about how to react. The adult startle response may be seen as the result of the completion of three developmental stages:

1. WITHDRAWAL REFLEX

This is an extreme reaction to "startle" resulting in immediate shut down or shock response—immobility, slowing of the heart rate, drop in blood pressure, cessation of breathing and extreme fear. A similar response can be seen in certain animals such as rabbits who "freeze" in one position when startled and remain motionless until the threat is removed.

It has been hypothesized that this early withdrawal response might be a precursor to the mammalian diving reflex, and the Fear Paralysis response described by Kaada (1988). Activation of the diving reflex results in immediate slowing down of the heart rate (bradycardia) and is thought to be a physiologically protective oxygen-conserving mechanism whereby the animal is kept alive during submergence by slowing down the metabolism and thereby protecting the brain from the deleterious effects of oxygen deprivation. Landsberg (1975) suggested that the diving reflex could act as *either* an oxygen-conserving mechanism *or* the start of a pathophysiological asphyxial response. In other words, if it is activated for too long, the results may be fatal. Kaada suggested that this might be an important factor in Sudden Infant Death Syndrome (SIDS).

Postural Control and the Coordination of Movement

Mature or conscious postural control is initiated in the motor cortex, but is dependent upon lower centers to coordinate and execute those movements in various stages of complexity. Starting from the lowest level:

1. Spinal Level — *simple reactions controlled only by nerve cells in the spinal cord which ensure that as one group of muscles contract, the opposing set relaxes.*

2. Brainstem and Midbrain — *act to keep muscles in a state of readi-ness maintaining muscle tone. The primitive and postural reflexes are mediated at the levels of the brainstem and midbrain.*

3. Basal Ganglia and Thalamus *coordinate each movement in cooperation with the cerebellum. The cerebellum then monitors and controls the progress of each movement.*

4. Cerebellum
Ultimately, the cerebellum is responsible for regulating the postural reflexes (Bloedel and Bracha 1997). Holt (1991) suggests that the cerebellum depends upon the postural reflexes to make fine motor skills automatic.

Uterine ───────▶

If this were the case, then it would be essential for nature to have installed an accessible "over-ride" mechanism. The Moro reflex might be just such an over-ride system. The characteristic of the withdrawal reaction is to shrink away from the stimulus and slow down the metabolism. The Moro reflex, on the other hand, activates the sympathetic nervous system which elicits immediate arousal. When fully developed, it belongs to the group of reflexes whose characteristic is to clasp or to embrace (rooting, suck, palmar and plantar reflexes). However, the Moro reflex develops in two stages: the first part emerges at 9-12 weeks after conception and comprises movement of the arms and legs outward and extension of the head (a withdrawal response) and after birth facilitates an intake of breath. It is only as the <u>second</u> part of the Moro reflex is developed (by 32 weeks after conception) that withdrawal is overcome by closing of the arms and legs, flexion of the head and, after birth, <u>release</u> of breath. The hypothesis mooted was that a full Moro reflex is necessary in the first months of life to inhibit the previous withdrawal response and protect the infant from an over-active withdrawal response to a startling situation.

If the earliest stage remains over-active, then the reflexes will operate in a reverse chain reaction, placing the infant at risk rather than protecting it from noxious stimuli. The withdrawal, Moro and adult startle reaction thus have the potential to operate in either direction in a chain response. If, however, the more mature response is fully developed, it should over-ride activation of the earlier one. This hypothesis is still to be proven.

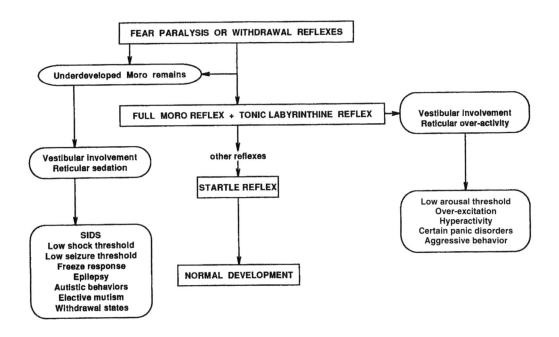

2. MORO REFLEX

Primitive

→

This is a primitive over-reaction to "startle," which results in stimulation of the sympathetic nervous system—increase in heart rate, immediate rise in blood pressure, rapid, shallow breathing, flushing of the face, accompanied by anger or distress. If for any reason the Moro reflex is only partially inhibited, the result can be defensive "body armoring" in an attempt to control the over-reaction through muscular tension. (Bennet 1988)

3. STRAUSS REFLEX

Postural

→

The adult startle reflex was described by Strauss in 1929 as "flexion of the legs and trunk, forward flexion of the head, raising and forward movement of the shoulders, forward raising and inward turning of the arms, pronation of the forearms, closing of the hands, lid blinking, facial grimacing and contraction of the abdominal muscles." It should develop at about four months of age as the Moro reflex is inhibited, although for a time both reactions may coexist. It is thought that cortical analysis of the required response is involved in the adult startle pattern, but is not a feature of the Moro reaction. Hence, the Moro individual reacts first and thinks afterwards.

Even in adults, all responses remain present, but once inhibited, the earlier ones should lie dormant, only to be awakened in situations of *extreme* danger.

POSTURAL CONTROL

Muscle tone: balance between flexor and extensor muscles.

Postnatal motor development takes place in a cephalo-caudal (head to toe) and proximo-distal (center outward) sequence. The development of postural reflexes should reflect this pattern. The first task a child must accomplish is mastery of head control and muscle tone, before further controlled voluntary movement can occur. Control is gained in the prone position before supine. By six weeks of age, the child can raise his head in line with his body when lying prone, and can hold it in that position for several seconds. By twelve weeks, he can lift his head well above the general body line and maintain it there for several minutes. By twelve weeks his legs are no longer flexed and his pelvis is flat on the surface when lying prone. By sixteen weeks he can press down with his forearms to lift his head and upper torso, stretching his limbs and "swim" in this position.

"Swimming" in prone position

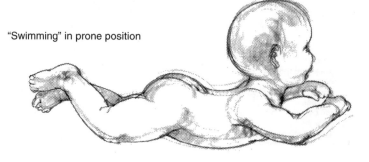

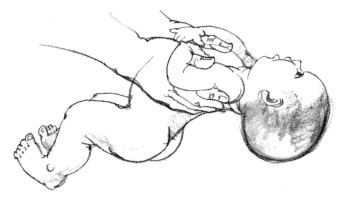

Head lag in supine position at 1 month of age

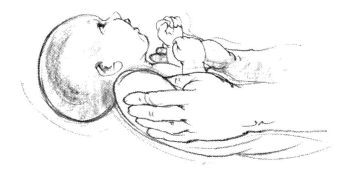

Head control to the midline at 3 months of age

RIGHTING REACTION

These are reactions to gravity which result from somatosensory, visual and proprioceptive influences acting *together* when the three inputs are available and functioning appropriately. With the exception of the oculo-headrighting reflex, for the most part they are integrated in the nuclei of the midbrain.

This gradual sequence of head control in the first 2-4 months of life heralds the development of the **oculo** and **labyrinthine headrighting reflexes**. Together these ensure that the head maintains a midline position (perpendicular to the ground when upright) despite movement of other parts of the body either actively or passively induced. The oculo-headrighting reflexes operate as a result of visual cues, while the labyrinthine headrighting reflexes are dependent upon vestibular information. The two should synchronize to supply accurate data upon which head position is adjusted. If they fail to develop fully, or only one develops adequately, balance, controlled eye movements and visual perception will all be impaired. Muscle tension in the neck and shoulder region combined with poor posture may therefore be symptoms of underdeveloped headrighting reflexes, as the 44 pairs of muscles in the neck responsible for holding the head up, fight to maintain head control without the support of automatic righting reactions.

There is a lag in attaining head control in the supine position which means that the infant is approximately 5 months of age before he can raise his head and hold it for some time above the level of the spine, in that position.

Headrighting reflexes in the older child—the head tilts in the opposite direction to the body.

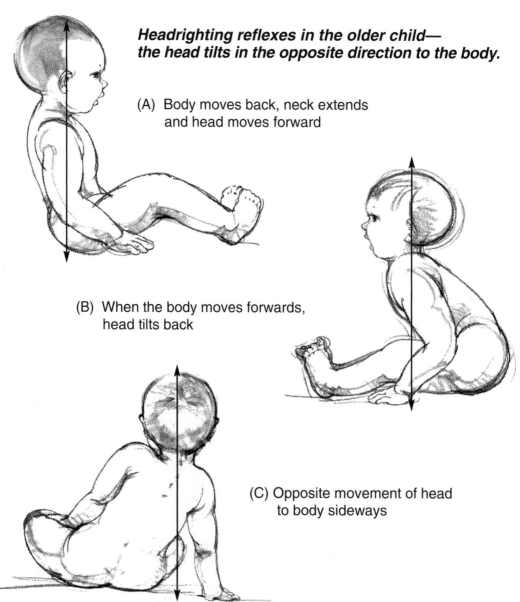

(A) Body moves back, neck extends and head moves forward

(B) When the body moves forwards, head tilts back

(C) Opposite movement of head to body sideways

LABYRINTHINE HEADRIGHTING REFLEX (LHRR)

The labyrinthine headrighting reflex is elicited by tilting of the body and/or stimulation of the otolithic organs. The reflex comprises compensatory contraction of the neck muscles to keep the head level.

OCULO-HEADRIGHTING REFLEX (OHRR)

Otoliths — minute crystalline particles suspended in a gelatinous mass into which the hair cells of the utricle and saccule of the inner ear project. They are under the influence of gravity and exert traction on the cilia of the hair cells during movements of the head and the body .

The oculo-headrighting reflex is initiated by visual cues and is dependent upon the functioning of the cerebral cortex. It maintains the head in a stable position and *the eyes fixed on visual targets* despite other movements of the body. This is necessary for fixation and sustained visual attention. The oculo-headrighting reflex may also be elicited by a combination of visual and vestibular stimulation, stretching of the neck muscles and/or movement of visual images on the retina.

In normal development, the visual abilities to fixate and to follow are enhanced as stability of head posture is achieved. If oculo-headrighting reflexes are underdeveloped, visual fixation and visual pursuit can be impaired. This can then affect reading ability, comprehension and spelling.

THE LANDAU REFLEX

The Landau reflex has a relatively short life span, emerging at the same time as the headrighting reflexes at 3-10 weeks of age, and being inhibited by the age of approximately three and a half years. The Landau reflex elicits extensor tone throughout the body in the prone position if the baby is suspended in the air with support under the stomach.

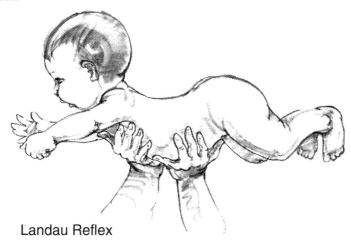

Landau Reflex

Neither the Landau nor the symmetrical tonic neck reflex is a true primitive or postural reflex. The Landau is not present at birth and therefore cannot be categorized as primitive. Neither remains present for the remainder of life and therefore is not a true postural reflex. Both seem to act as important "bridge" reflexes which have an inhibitory effect upon the tonic labyrinthine reflex, strengthen muscle tone and develop vestibulo-ocular motor skills.

Development of the Landau reflex helps to increase muscle tone when prone. Simultaneously it acts as an inhibitory influence upon the tonic labyrinthine reflex (TLR) forwards, increasing headrighting, and muscle tone in the torso. It enables the child to elevate not only the head but also the chest, and is an important prerequisite for more advanced movements involving the arms and hands later on. At three and a half years of age, by which time the child should be secure as a mobile biped, the Landau reflex should no longer be necessary. Its continued presence in later life suggests underlying primitive reflex activity, and will affect development of balance and of voluntary alteration of muscle tone in rapidly changing conditions, e.g. a child may run with stiff awkward movement in the lower half of the body, and find hopping, skipping and jumping difficult as he cannot flex the leg muscles at will.

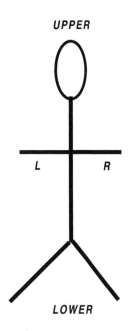

UPPER

L   R

LOWER

THE AMPHIBIAN REFLEX

The amphibian reflex should develop at 4-6 months of life, first in prone, then in supine. Elevation of the pelvis elicits automatic flexion from the hip to affect the knee on the same side.

Flexion of one leg irrespective of head position permits an increase in mobility and marks an important stage for the development of crawling on the tummy. Hitherto, flexion or extension of the legs bilaterally has been dependent upon head position and has been determined by the activities of the asymmetrical tonic neck reflex (ATNR). The amphibian reflex thus denotes significant inhibition of the ATNR. Freedom from this constraint permits the independent movement of the legs and arms essential for crawling, creeping and gross muscle coordination later on and enables the child to move one quadrant of the body independently of the other three.

An <u>underdeveloped</u> amphibian reflex will impede cross pattern crawling and creeping and may contribute to hypertonus in later life thus interfering with activities dependent upon gross muscle coordination e.g. physical education, sports, etc. Total lack of an amphibian reflex suggests uninhibited primitive reflexes, particularly the asymmetrical tonic neck reflex (ATNR) and the tonic labyrinthine reflex (TLR).

SEGMENTAL ROLLING REFLEXES

The segmental rolling reflexes are a later modification of the "neck on body and body righting reactions." Whereas the neck and body righting reactions align the trunk with the head when either is rotated or turned, the segmental rolling reflexes are strictly rotational responses.

The body on body righting reaction occur if the infant is laid on its side and pressure is applied to the side of the body. This initiates reflex righting of the body (even if the labyrinths have been destroyed). If the head is turned the body will follow in line with the head in a "log roll."

The neck on body righting reactions act if the head is righted but the body is tilted out of alignment. This results in the thorax righting and initiates a wave of stretch reflexes that pass down the body, righting the abdomen and the legs.

The segmental rolling reflexes develop at two key positions in the body: the shoulders and the hips. Movement starts at the head, then follows to the shoulders, thorax and pelvis or vice versa.

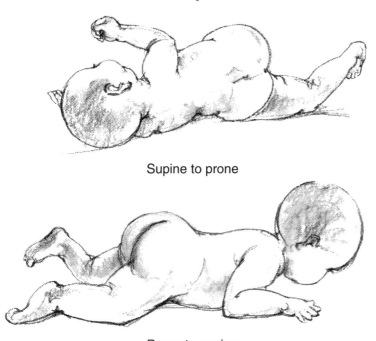

Supine to prone

Prone to supine

These reflexes start to emerge at 6 months of age to allow rolling, first from supine to prone at 6 months, then from prone to supine at 8-10 months, followed by sitting, four point kneeling and eventually standing. As the child becomes practiced and adept at these activities, the reflex becomes redundant for progress from lying to standing, but should remain through life to facilitate changing positions and to give fluidity to movements such as running, jumping, skiing, etc.

EQUILIBRIUM REACTIONS

Equilibrium reactions affect our ability to maintain balance, particularly moving balance. They are neces- sary for a child to maintain control of movement while in action (running, jumping, hopping). Children who lack equilib- rium reactions tend to be clumsy, fall over more often than their peers and have dificulty with movements which require sudden shifts in direction. (Pyfer & Johnson 1981)

The establishment of postural righting reactions is only the beginning of postural control. Once the righting reactions are operating, equilibrium reactions start to develop from circa nine months of age. Equilibrium reactions are elicited by stimulation of the labyrinths; they are compensatory in nature in response to changes in the center of gravity, and they should become available to modify the patterns of righting reactions.

Equilibrium reactions are primarily protective in nature; they occur in response to a sudden alteration in position or when balance is lost. They are dependent upon visual stimulation, and it has been suggested that they are linked to the adult "startle" or Strauss reflex. (Fiorentino 1981)

The parachute reflex may be elicited if the infant is held in the air and then tilted forward toward the ground. The arms extend as if to protect the head and trunk from the full force of impact. If the infant is held upright and dropped rapidly toward the ground, the lower limbs first extend, tense then abduct. The reflex's value is a protective one.

At approximately six months of age the sideways parachute or "propping" reflex also emerges. This is essential if a child is to learn to sit, since it provides for any loss of balance in the sitting position by compensatory movement of the arm on the side to which the child is falling, "propping" the trunk and preventing the infant from toppling over. This reflex should be present during the child's early attempts at standing, cruising and walking.

Combined effects of immature reflexes

If a higher level of response is unavailable, an organism will respond regressively with the next most mature response it can muster. If, for example, a child has under-developed righting or equilibrium reactions there is no effective mechanism as protection against falling when balance is lost—loss of balance may then activate the Moro reflex as the final defense available because higher systems have failed.

Lack of gravitational security (Ayres 1989) can result in generalized insecurity and greater susceptibility to anxiety — both often typical in children with coordination problems and poor postural control. The effect may also be seen in adolescents and adults who appear to have compensated for underlying postural problems, but who start to experience emotional difficulties when placed under increased academic stress. These may be the youngsters who manifest learning related problems for the first time when they reach higher education, when the education system is less structured and greater flexibility in learning styles is required.

Whereas there is documented evidence that retained primitive reflexes underlie difficulties in the learning of basic skills such as reading, writing and copying, less attention has been paid to the role of postural reflexes in providing a functional link between postural control, cognitive functioning and academic performance.

Dr. Lawrence J. Beuret, who works in Chicago with adolescents and young adults who have Neuro-Developmental problems, has found that members of this older age group sometimes present a profile in which the primitive reflexes have been inhibited but the postural reflexes have not developed fully. These youngsters *appear* to have compensated well and therefore have not been identified as having a problem until relatively late in development —sometimes well into adolesence or beyond. Unfortunately, these are the children who would have benefited from motor training or sensory integration intervention at an earlier age. The specific symptoms this group shows are typically problems in:

- Adaptation
- Applying known concepts (problem solving)
- Linking
- Multi-processing
- Sequencing
- Coping with large volumes of information
  (information overload)

All of the above are skills which become essential at higher levels of education.

Additional related problems in this older age group may include:

- History of fine motor disturbances
- Low energy levels which mimic depression but which do not respond to medication
- Lack of torso flexibility (trunkal integration)
- Difficulty carrying out complex movement patterns such as those required in martial arts or dance routines. Often they will comment on having to "think through" each movement sequence and have difficulty adapting to rapid changes in routine.

The effect on a child of having underdeveloped postural reflexes is the environmental and social equivalent of having an under-developed vocabulary. Often an individual can cope as long as the rules remain the same and it is possible to use previously learned skills. If the rules required by a situation change, such children are forced to "learn and practice" the new rules because they are not able to adapt and change to meet the altered circumstances. This can result in "awkwardness," feelings of personal and social inadequacy and increased propensity to suffer from anxiety.

Development of the Reflex System

Vulnerability to any invasive outside stimuli.

Automatic reaction involving the whole body

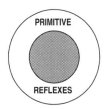

Involuntary reactions to external stimuli or motor activity. Auto-matic stereotyped response— allow no leeway for varation or choice of action.

Vulnerability and over-reaction —limited systems of response.

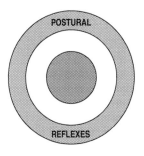

Automatic reactions for the main-tenance of balance, stability and flexibility throughout the body.

Provide the foundations for voluntary, adaptive responses to environmental changes.

REFLEX MATURATION — A CONTINUING PROCESS

There are many other reflexes in addition to the postural reflexes outlined previously, which have an impact upon both motor and sensory functioning. One example of a later, non-postural reflex is the **Acoustic Stapedius Reflex**. The stapedius muscle of the inner ear is attached to the stapes and it is the smallest muscle in the human body. If there is a loud noice, the acoustic stapedius reflex should activate involuntary contraction of the stapedius muscle immediately after the sound (usually noises louder than 80-90 decibels). The effect is to dampen the sound that is actually heard by as much as 20 decibels or more, thereby protecting the inner ear from noise damage. The reflex should also occur just before a person vocalizes to reduce interference from the sound of one's own voice.

The contraction of the stapedius pulls the ossicles--the tiny bones in the ear--away from the eardrum and so lessens the impact of sound vibrations.

The nerve that controls this muscle mingles with fibers of the facial nerve. Thus it interacts with the nerves that control facial expression and those that bring information from the skin of the external ear. (Kandel 1991)

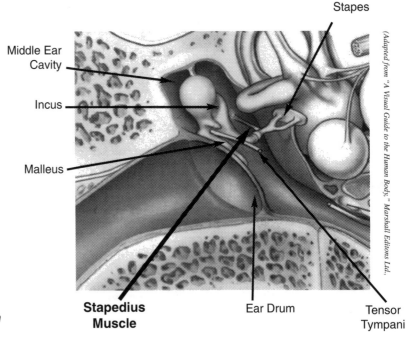

Stapes

Middle Ear Cavity

Incus

Malleus

Stapedius Muscle

Ear Drum

Tensor Tympani

(Adapted from "A Visual Guide to the Human Body," Marshall Editions Ltd.)

The acoustic stapedius reflex starts to operate between 2 and 4 months of age, at the same time as the Moro reflex is being inhibited. The hypersensitivity to sound observed in many children and adults who still have traces of a Moro reflex might be because the continued presence of the Moro reflex has prevented the acoustic stapedius reflex from developing fully. Equally, lack of an acoustic stapedius reflex might activate a Moro startle response because there is no adequate protection against loud noise. This might also be a factor in children who seem to be abnormally timid, who avoid situations where there are loud noises. They hate balloons—they might pop—and detest fireworks. Often they talk as if they were afraid of their own voice. Certain methods of sound therapy probaby help to develop this reflex and may be one reason why some autistic children respond well to Auditory Integrative Training. *(see Chapter 4)*

Reflexes and sensory processing cannot be separated. The following diagrams illustrate just some of the connections between primitive and postural reflexes and the senses.

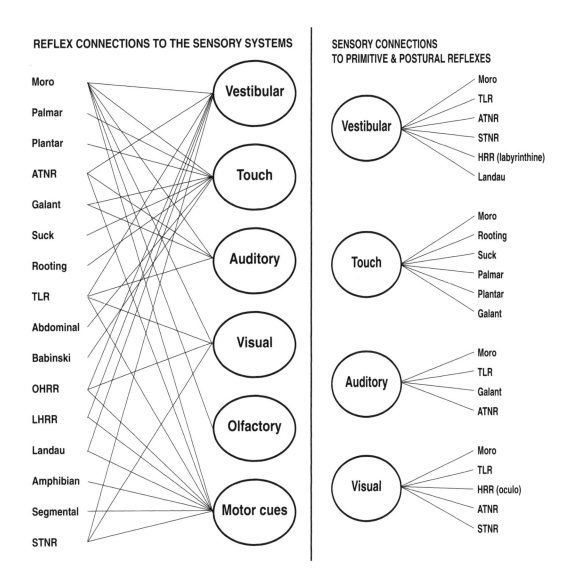

In functional terms, the postural reflexes form part of a main highway of connections from the motor cortex to the muscles. If part of that highway is still under construction, it can interfere with rapid progress of information along that route. Alternative routes can be used, but the alternative routes may be neither as efficient nor as direct as the main pathway.

Chapter 3

BRAIN
DEVELOPMENT

Absent or underdeveloped postural reflexes have long been accepted as contributory factors in coordination problems and associated disorders, such as dyspraxia, "clumsy child" syndrome, apraxia, etc. With this in mind, motor training programs have been devised to encourage the development of postural reflexes, and thus improve coordination and balance. Some of these, such as what has become known as the Doman-Delacato program, are based on the concept that brain organization has an impact on learning problems and can be changed by repeating early developmental movements.

> *Glenn Doman and Carl Delacato have long since gone in their separate directions. Their techniques have evolved and improved over the years and their methods should not be evaluated by what they advocated twenty-five years ago. Carl Delacato has also pioneered in the treatment of autistic children.*

The techniques employed in sensory integration (A. Jean Ayres) are based upon the concept that stimulation of the postural reflexes through specific physical exercises can encourage the development of more mature patterns of response and will also suppress underlying primitive reflex activity. General improvement in balance and coordination demonstrate the value of such programs, particularly where the source of the problem lies in lack of postural reflexes with only minimal primitive reflex activity still present.

If the primitive reflexes are still strong, however, stimulation of postural reflexes alone will rarely reap concomitant changes in the areas of fine muscle coordination, oculomotor functioning, perceptual processing and academic performance. This may be because, while motor training programs strengthen postural control, they fail to inhibit those retained primitive reflexes which continue to impede the processing of information in the brain. In order to understand why this may be the case, we need to examine some of the mechanisms within the brain and how they develop during the first year of life.

Establishing a hierarchy

The brain comprises many separate entities which are all interlinked and dependent upon each other. At birth, connections to the superficial layers of the cortex are only tenuously made. In the first few months and years of life the developing child must form millions of new connections between nerve cells which will provide a network of communication or neural circuitry of almost unimaginable complexity upon which future behavior and learning will be based. The layering of the connections between motor areas is sometimes viewed as a hierarchy of systems involving multiple levels of control.

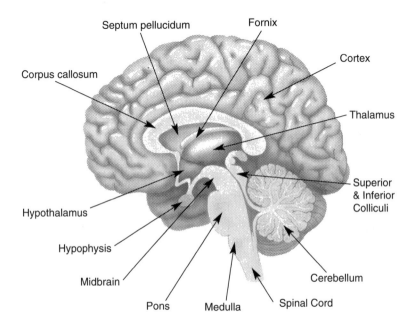

*Brainstem —
the range of bulges
that forms the central
core of the brain
running from the top
of the spinal cord
into the middle of the
brain. It comprises
the medulla, pons
and midbrain.*

Starting from the lowest level: **Spinal Level**
Spinal mechanisms provide a point of contact between the nervous system and the muscles. Simple reflexive movements controlled only by nerve cells in the spinal cord ensure that as one group of muscles contract, the opposing set relax. An example of a spinal reflex can be seen in the case of the sea slug which reacts automatically with a withdrawal response if an unexpected blast of water is aimed at its abdominal cavity. Spinal reflexes can be modified by higher levels in the brain.

Brainstem
The brainstem is situated at the head of the spinal column and houses the nerve pathways which carry impulses between the brain and the body. It is part of the central nervous system (CNS) and is responsible for the neurons which control heart beat, blood pressure, breathing and also the signals to swallow, laugh, sneeze, etc. It forms the evolutionary core or primitive site, which is shared by man, fish and reptile. The

function it fulfills is so fundamental that injury to the core of the brainstem results in death. The brainstem also contains the point at which the nerve tracts between brain and the body cross over and change course to the opposite side. The brainstem includes the pons and medulla oblongata. Primitive reflexes are mediated at the level of the brainstem, while the postural reflexes with the exception of the oculo-headrighting reflex are controlled from the midbrain. Linked to the brainstem is the vital reticular formation, which is responsible for maintaining consciousness and arousal.

CORTICAL CONTROL

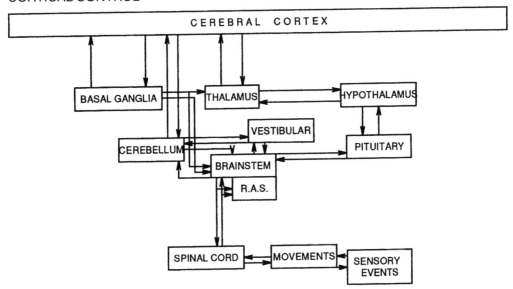

The reticular activating system (R.A.S.) is like the brain's own alarm clock, monitoring sensory signals and passing them through to alert or "calm down" according to the circumstances. It plays an important part in maintaining consciousness and in the regulation of the sleep-wake cycle and therefore also affects waking alertness and the ability to pay attention.

R.A.S. —
A complex network of nerve fibers, occupying the central core of the brainstem, that function in wakefulness and alertness

Both conscious and automatic control of the sensory motor system depends on the constant, though fluctuating, interactions between all the different centers —including the cerebellum— that comprise the central nervous system.

The thalamus is a twin-lobed mass of nerve cells at the top of the brainstem. It acts as an important relay station for sensory and motor fibers. It both sends and receives impulses from the cerebellum, reticular system, neural ganglia and the cortex. All of the senses with the exception of smell are filtered through the thalamus before they reach their specialized regions in the cortex, and it therefore plays a vital role in the potential interpretation of sensory stimuli.

Autopsy studies of subjects with Dyslexia as well as brain activation studies of living subjects have implicated dysfunction in large areas of the brain, some of which are concerned with language, others with general sound processing. Animal models indicate that induction of cortical malformations (possibly during fetal development or at birth) such as those seen in the brains of subjects with Dyslexia can lead to sound processing anomalies and anatomic changes in the thalamus. These subtle changes in the structure of the thalamus then have an impact upon the processing of sensory information. (Galaburda 2001)

The **hypothalamus** is situated slightly below the thalamus and acts as the synthesizer of the hormones involved in temperature control, water balance, hunger and sexual behavior. These hormones are then funneled into the pituitary gland where they are stored or released into the bloodstream. These two centers together with the hippocampus and amygdala are labeled the seat of the limbic system, which man has in common with other mammals. It is from the limbic system that feelings of passion, drive, fear, anger and grief are all generated. If the brainstem represents survival, then it is the midbrain and the limbic system that represent what we call instinct, and which largely controls our metabolism, our feelings (physiological sensations of emotion) and our metabolic reactions to the outside world. The limbic system is also involved in the laying down of memories which may be one reason why children seem to learn better when they relate physically and emotionally to the material. It is also why the memory of past traumatic events can reawaken the physical sensations of fear and distress associated with the original event.

It has been suggested (Gaddes 1980) that some behavior results directly from reflexive or spontaneous stimulation of the hypothalamus and related structures, combined with inhibitory learned processes emanating from the cerebral cortex. *"Too much hypothalamic stimulation with too little cortical (or intellectual) control presumably results in the socially obnoxious child who disregards the rights and wishes of others. The reverse pattern may result in the overcontrolled, inhibited, unimaginative child."* This sounds remarkably similar to the two profiles which are characteristic of the Moro directed child described in Chapter 1.

Basal Ganglia— three small masses of nerve tissue involved in the subconscious regulation of movements

The basal ganglia are a group of nuclei at the base of the cerebral cortex which help regulate body movements. The basal ganglia are responsible for the organization of involuntary and semivoluntary activity, upon which consciously willed movements are superimposed. They receive input from the cerebral cortex and then influence movement by affecting the output of the motor cortex. The basal ganglia and the cerebellum are involved in various aspects of planning and monitoring of movements but have no outputs of their own to the spinal cord. They are prominently involved in adjusting ongoing movements and should maintain the balance between inhibitory and facilitating influences. When a particular part of the basal ganglia (the striatum) is damaged, such as occurs in Parkinson's disease, inhibition of involuntary movement is impaired and continuous tremor is present when the patient is at rest. Activities which at first need practice should eventually be absorbed into the automatic repertoire of the basal ganglia together with the cerebellum. Learning to play the piano, learning to drive a car or ride a bicycle, would fall into that category.

The Cerebellum

Connected to the brainstem, but not a part of it, is the cerebellum. Its name literally means "the little brain."

While it is the cerebral cortex that enables us to perform all the higher functions which are unique to mankind, it is the cerebellum which governs man's every movement. Although it can initiate nothing by itself, the cerebellum monitors impulses from the motor centers in the brain and from the nerve endings in the muscles. Incoming impulses outnumber efferent impulses 3:1 for it is the cerebellum's job to sift and to fine tune relevant information. Impulses to the cerebellum are directed from the vestibular system, the eyes and the muscle joints of the lower limbs and trunk. Ultimately, the cerebellum is responsible for regulating the postural reflexes and muscle tone (Bloedal and Brachfa 1997), and in this way, for maintaining the body's equilibrium.[Note 1]

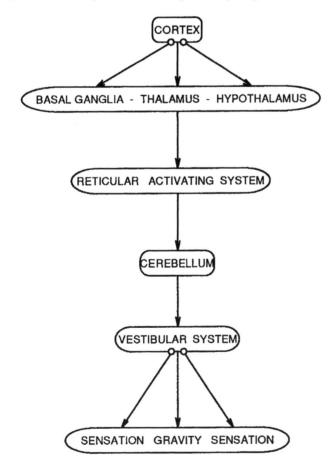

The Cerebellum and Development

The cerebellum is situated at the back of the brain, above the brainstem and below the cerebral cortex. Like the neocortex, it is more highly developed in man than in any other species and it accounts for 11% of the entire brain's weight. From birth to four years of age it grows at a faster rate than the cortex, attaining 80% of its adult size by two years of age and completing a major period of myelination by four years of age. It continues to develop at a slower rate up to 15 years of age and beyond.

Its period of most rapid growth and maturation occurs at the time that early motor patterns are being learned. As early motor patterns are learned and practiced, they are filed away in the basal ganglia and cerebellum, to be accessed when required. The cerebellum assimilates the actions involved in complex and habitually used movements, and then releases sequences of movements on command, modifying parts of the sequence to match output to intent. This is the motoric equivalent of building up a vocabulary. The cerebellum is particularly involved in the *learning* stages of a new skill, but as a child becomes more adept at a skill, less cerebellar activity is involved.

The cerebellum learns by **doing**; practice improves performance as a result of synaptic connections being repeatedly fired and the involved neurons adapting their function to become more efficient.

Archicerebellum— ancient cerebellum.

Paleocerebellum— old cerebellum.

Neocerebellum— new cerebellum.

Similar to the brain as a whole, the cerebellum is organized in three layers. At the base is the **archicerebellum**. This is an evolutionary outgrowth of the vestibular system, from where certain fibers pass directly to the cerebellar cortex, while the majority relay information via the vestibular nuclei and the reticular activating system in the brainstem. The **paleocerebellum** receives action potentials from the skin, joints and primary endings of the neuro-muscular spindles (tactile and proprioceptive connections). The **neocerebellum** has developed together with the cerebral cortex in mammals. It has achieved its greatest size in primates, of which the evolutionary most recent part, the neodendate of the dentate nucleus, is present only in man. The neocerebellum plays a major part in the control of hand and mouth movements and is therefore also involved in speech, articulation and the fine control of manipulative skills, of which handwriting is one. [(Note 2)]

Dysdiadochokinesia— difficulty with rapid, alternate movements.

INPP has found that a high percentage of children who have abnormal primitive and postural reflexes also demonstrate difficulties with dysdiadochokinesia of the fingers, hands and feet, a skill which comes under the regulation of the cerebellum.

Development of Cerebellar Connections

When a child is born, the different regions of the brain are functional but not fully linked. How does the young child develop and integrate these systems in the first years of life? In prenatal development it is the vestibular system which is remarkable for its precocious development, being in place at eight weeks after conception, functional at 16 weeks, and myelinated at the time of birth. It is the only one of the sensory systems to be mature at birth with both its afferent and efferent cerebellar linkages, but in the first few months of life it must learn to interact effectively with the other sensory systems (touch, vision and hearing) which mature rapidly from the time of birth to form major connections to the cerebral cortex.

ORGANIZATION & MAJOR CONNECTIONS IN THE CEREBELLUM

Phylogenetic	Major Connections	Type of Function
Archicerebellum	Vestibular	Posture (subconscious)
Paleocerebellum	Spinal Cord Sensory	Progressive movement eg. walking, running, etc.
Neocerebellum	Cerebral Cortex via Pons	Fine muscle coordination, particularly of the hands and mouth.
Dentate Nucleus	Association Cortex	—word association —mental imagery of movement sequences (ideation) —practice related learning —error detection —judging time intervals & velocity of moving stimuli —rapidly shifting attention between sensory modalities —cognitive operations in 3D space

(Results shown on PET scans, Leiner, Leiner and Dow, 1993)

The archicerebellum matures early in fetal life but it will take until at least 15 months to four years of age for the first stage of neocerebellar connections to the cerebral cortex to be laid down.

Reflex movements provide a child with its earliest movement vocabulary.

One of the ways a child learns to calibrate these different systems is through *movement;* through utilization and practice of movement patterns over and over again. First, through spontaneous and reflexive movements and later through developing voluntary control over an increasing range of movements and postural control. Movement feeds information to the brain, helping to develop a sense of body map, of spatial awareness and body schema in relation to the self and to the environment. The dual processes of maturation and environmental opportunity operate in concert to facilitate this process. The cerebellum can then utilize the information to modify and refine subsequent motor activity. A reflex stimulation/inhibition program may improve cerebellar functioning by maturing the postural reflex system through which the cerebellum operates. [Notes 3, 4]

The smooth operation of the motor system is dependent upon the entire central nervous system, both motor and sensory. Voluntary and semi-voluntary movement develop through practice, but are not possible without pre-existing postural patterns which are already established by the basal-reticular system. As the child approaches maturity, the order of command should function from the top downward with the cerebral cortex influencing and modifying the action of the basal ganglia, which in turn modifies centers of the brainstem, then modifying the cord reflexes. At every level there is a feedback of information to the centers, and the cerebellum acts as the vital monitor in this feedback network. Dysfunction at any level releases centers below from the influences of those above. Equally, failure of lower centers to be inhibited will prevent higher centers from maintaining control. The chain of command should resemble the diagram in Fig. 8.

FEEDBACK OF INFORMATION

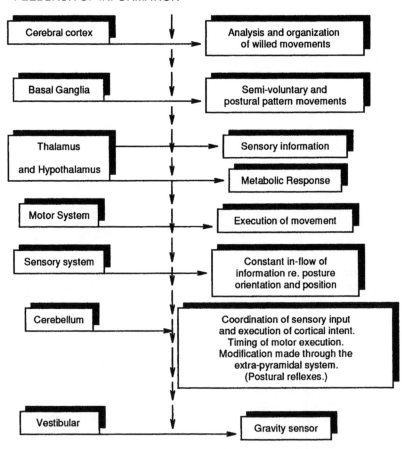

Cerebellar damage can cause paralysis in affected regions of the body. Cerebellar dysfunction can result in clumsiness affecting visualmotor performance and manual dexterity. Hence the cerebellum used to be known as "the patron saint of the clumsy child." (Restak 1991) As the regulator of the postural reflexes, cerebellar-dependent functions will be profoundly affected if the postural reflexes fail to develop. Equally, cerebellar dysfunction may prevent the development of postural reflexes. The

cerebellum also plays an important role in sequential and rote learning, and in short term memory. This may be one reason why medication aimed at the cerebellum and the vestibular apparatus (Levinson 1984) dramatically improves the performance of some dyslexic children.

Finally, at the top of the brain pyramid is the cerebral cortex, comprising two hemispheres which are linked together by the corpus callosum. Although some tasks are shared by both hemispheres, the left and right side of the cerebral cortex have specialized functions to perform, but are dependent upon each other for the execution of those tasks, hence the significance of the corpus callosum between them. The corpus callosum contains millions of nerve fibers which facilitate communication and instantaneous feedback from one side of the brain to the other.

If, for example, the two sides of the cortex were chemically or surgically separated, and the patient asked to pick out two previously identified faces in a large crowd, each side would use a different method. The left side of the brain would laboriously search every face one by one in logical sequence until it found the face it was looking for. The right brain would scan the sea of faces until it alighted on the target, but the owner of the brain could not tell us their name, since connection to the language center in the left hemisphere has been cut. Communication between the two sides is obviously of vital importance.

One of the major differences between men and women can be seen here, as the corpus callosum develops to be 40% larger in women than in men. This may go some way to explaining man's tendency to be more "single minded" in his approach to tackling problems, while the woman can be aware of a number of factors simultaneously. It is in the cortex that information passed on from all the other brain centers becomes conscious, and on the basis of cortical analysis, decisions for action will be made. The cortex should be the seat of intellect, of decision and of controlled response, but it can only do its job easily and effectively if the reflexive action of the lower centers are integrated at the correct time, in a hierarchical sequence.

The corpus callosum also seems to act as a screening device, at times shielding information between the two sides of the cortex. It should be capable of either transmitting or inhibiting exchange of information.

If the corpus callosum fails to *pass* information fluently from one side to the other, the child may have difficulty decoding certain types of information, linking known facts to new situations and solving problems. One side of the brain may not be given the opportunity to recognize it knows the answer or to communicate the relevant information to the other side of the brain. This is sometimes a problem in children diagnosed with Attention Deficit Disorder (ADD).

If the corpus callosum fails to *inhibit* the transmission of information from one side of the brain to the other, it can result in too much interference and lack of hemispheric specialization. Exercises to develop bilateral integration may help this type of problem (see Chapter 5).

HEMISPHERIC SPECIALIZATION

In addition to having specific skills, the right hemisphere of the cortex seems to play an important part in the learning of new tasks. In a sense it is the "practice ground" for newly acquired skills, which will then defer to the left hemisphere to apply dissection, logic and detail. When a certain level of understanding or attainment has been reached, one side of the brain can become the "specialist" for that task.

> *"In initial reading, the balance of brain activity favors the right hemisphere, whereas advanced readers favor the left hemisphere. Thus, there is a moment in the learning-to-read process at which the balance in the brain tips from right to left at approximately the age of $6^{1}/_{2}$-$7^{1}/_{2}$ years."* **Bakker (1990)**

This is the same age at which a major period of myelination and "linking" takes place between the vestibular apparatus, the cerebellum and the corpus callosum. It is then no quantum leap to suppose that a child's reading readiness is closely linked to his neuro-developmental age. Developmental age may not necessarily be parallel with chronological age and the teaching methods should be chosen taking the child's developmental stage into consideration.

Right hemisphere reading is based on visio-spatial and holistic skills, e.g. whole words, or "look-say" method.

Left hemisphere reading involves decoding of individual symbols, word building from letters, and phonetics based skills.

Victims of left hemisphere damage demonstrate severe speech and language problems. One young man who had been in a ghastly car accident in his early 20's and suffered severe left hemisphere damage as a result, was able to describe what it felt like for him: *"I no longer see sound as I used to. Sound for me is a flat map; there are no hills and valleys although I know there once were. I know what I want to say but the words are like Everest and I cannot see the top."* His speech was flat, monotone, stuttering and without cadence. He was attempting to use the sublanguage center of the right hemisphere to communicate, and the result was like that of an adult making first attempts at a foreign language. Many children who are left-ear dominant demonstrate some form of language difficulty either in speech or written spelling. Galaburda's (1978) research on the brains of dyslexics shows that a high percentage have abnormally small left hemispheres, suggesting either lack of left hemisphere development from the outset, or underdevelopment through lack of use.

> *In the Far East, where the written language is based on pictograms, dyslexia barely exists. Much of Eastern philosophy is also based on right hemisphere thinking, i.e. the ability for past, present and future to coexist simultaneously. When we dream, we also do this, so that logically disconnected events can be brought together and viewed through visio-spatial, holistic representation.*

Dyslexics appear to favor right hemisphere methods of learning. When reading, writing and spelling, they have difficulty applying left hemisphere techniques. This is unfortunate, because such usage might further enhance left hemisphere maturation. [Note 5]

CEREBRUM

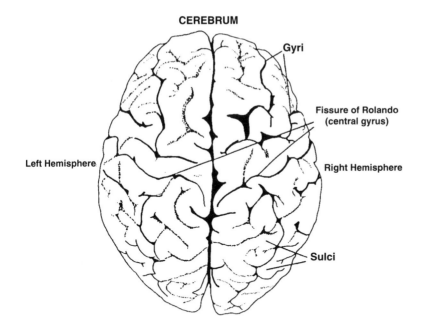

Gyri

Fissure of Rolando
(central gyrus)

Left Hemisphere

Right Hemisphere

Sulci

Unilaterality:
dominance of one side
of the cortex over the
other.

Continued presence of the asymmetrical tonic neck reflex (ATNR) interferes with unilaterality of brain function. (Gesell & Ames 1947, Telleus, C.1980) This results in homolateral patterns of movement and causes a midline barrier to cross-pattern movements of the body, and also slows speed of transmission within the brain.

Homolateral:
one side of the body at
a time. i.e. arm and leg
on one side of the body
move together. In the
adult this may cause a
soldier to be unable to
march, or the dancing
partner to seem to
have two left feet.

Difficulties with dysdiadochokinesia are symptomatic of lack of cerebral dominance, or put another way, until the cerebellum has mastered control of fine muscle movements so that the child can perform the finger-opposition test without difficulty, independent movement of each side of the body has not been established, and cerebral dominance has not occurred.

Dysdiadochokinesia:
difficulty with rapid
alternate movement,
e.g. fine muscle move-
ment in the hands,
finger or feet. This
will affect handicraft
activities and may also
be linked to speech
defects.

In the cerebellum the greatest period of growth and of maturation occurs between birth and 15 months of age, just the period when the adjustments from primitive reflex to postural control are being made. Maturation continues at a slower rate until the age of seven or eight years, when the final "linking" takes place between the vestibular apparatus, the cerebellum and the corpus callosum. It is generally accepted that occasional letter, number and word reversals in reading and writing are normal until the age of approximately eight years. This is the time when this final linking should have taken place. Continued reversal after this age may not be merely symptomatic of a dyslexic type of problem, but may also be suggestive of vestibular/cerebellar immaturity with implications for many other areas of functioning. Lack of postural reflexes would confirm this diagnosis.

BIRTH TO FOUR MONTHS OF AGE

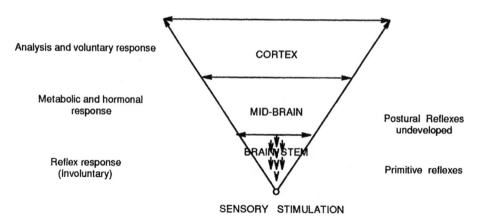

Analysis and voluntary response

Metabolic and hormonal response

Reflex response (involuntary)

CORTEX

MID-BRAIN

BRAIN STEM

SENSORY STIMULATION

Postural Reflexes undeveloped

Primitive reflexes

FOUR TO TWELVE MONTHS OF AGE

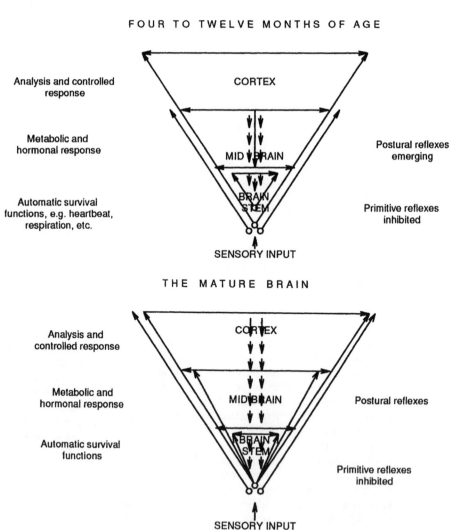

Analysis and controlled response

Metabolic and hormonal response

Automatic survival functions, e.g. heartbeat, respiration, etc.

CORTEX

MID BRAIN

BRAIN STEM

SENSORY INPUT

Postural reflexes emerging

Primitive reflexes inhibited

THE MATURE BRAIN

Analysis and controlled response

Metabolic and hormonal response

Automatic survival functions

CORTEX

MID BRAIN

BRAIN STEM

SENSORY INPUT

Postural reflexes

Primitive reflexes inhibited

The term "triune brain" (MacLean, P. 1979) describes the brain as being divided into three levels. Each level embodies or represents a stage in evolution. The brainstem symbolizes the "reptilian brain," because it is shared by all vertebrates from reptile to man. In his early weeks of life, the neonate is a totally brainstem dominated creature, and the movements that he makes are reptilian in character —head lift, squirming and rolling in a gravity bound world. The midbrain represents MacLean's "mammalian brain" and takes the young infant through the stages of rolling, crawling, sitting, creeping and standing. Finally, the cortex takes control, enabling us to stand and to move with independent use of the hands, and eventually to grow into rational, logical linguistic and altruistic human beings. All levels remain within us, but lower brain regions should not remain predominant. If they do, they will prevent the final stage of cortical control from being acquired completely.

Fiorentino (1981) linked the primitive and postural reflexes to three stages in the development of mobility —**apedal, quadruped** and **bipedal**— each one signifying a new stage in the recapitulation of our evolutionary heritage and the active involvement of higher systems of the brain.

LEVELS OF DEVELOPMENT

3. Bipedal — initiated at the **cortical** level involving many other centers including the basal ganglia and the cerebellum. Equilibrium reactions develop when muscle tone is normal to facilitate body adaptation in response to change in the center of gravity.

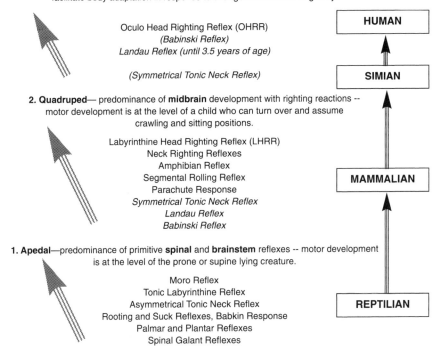

Oculo Head Righting Reflex (OHRR)
(Babinski Reflex)
Landau Reflex (until 3.5 years of age)

(Symmetrical Tonic Neck Reflex)

| HUMAN |
| SIMIAN |

2. Quadruped— predominance of **midbrain** development with righting reactions -- motor development is at the level of a child who can turn over and assume crawling and sitting positions.

Labyrinthine Head Righting Reflex (LHRR)
Neck Righting Reflexes
Amphibian Reflex
Segmental Rolling Reflex
Parachute Response
Symmetrical Tonic Neck Reflex
Landau Reflex
Babinski Reflex

| MAMMALIAN |

1. Apedal—predominance of primitive **spinal** and **brainstem** reflexes -- motor development is at the level of the prone or supine lying creature.

Moro Reflex
Tonic Labyrinthine Reflex
Asymmetrical Tonic Neck Reflex
Rooting and Suck Reflexes, Babkin Response
Palmar and Plantar Reflexes
Spinal Galant Reflexes

| REPTILIAN |

It is through the process of primitive reflex inhibition and then postural reflex development, that the infant recapitulates evolution. [Note 6]

HIERARCHICAL CONNECTIONS BETWEEN THE BRAIN, REFLEXES AND FUNCTIONING

Integrated In	Reflex	Stimulus	Response	Receptor
Spinal Cord and medulla	Stretch reflexes	Stretch	Contraction of muscle	Muscle Spindle
Spinal Cord	Positive supporting reaction (magnet)	Contact on sole of foot/body (or upper-hand body)	Foot extended to support	Proprioceptive flexors
Spinal Cord	Negative supporting reaction	Stretch	Release of positive support reaction	Proprioceptive extensors
Medulla	Tonic Labyrinthine Reflex	Gravity	Contraction of limb extensor (hands/knees table position)	
Medulla	Tonic Neck Reflexes (ATNR STNR)	Head turned: 1 to side 2 up 3 down	1 Extension of limbs on side to which head is turned 2 Legs flex 3 Arms flex	
Midbrain	Labyrinthine Head Righting Reflexes	Gravity	Head alignment	Otolithic organs
Midbrain	Neck Righting Reflexes	Stretch of neck muscles	Righting of thorax, shoulders, then pelvis	Muscle spindle
Midbrain	Body on head righting reflexes	Pressure on side of body	Righting of head	Exteroceptors
Midbrain	Body on body righting	Pressure on side of body	Righting of body even when head held sideways	Exteroceptors
Cerebral Cortex	Optical head righting reflexes	Visual cues	Righting of head	Eyes
Cerebral Cortex	Placing reactions	Various visual, exteroceptive and proprioceptive cues	Foot placed on supporting surface in position to support body	Various
Cerebral Cortex	Hopping reactions	Lateral displacement while standing	Hops, maintaining limbs in place to support body	Muscle spindles

Table adapted from Ganong (1997) and Galley & Forster (1982)

Chapter 4

THE SENSES

Long before a child ever reaches school age, he has begun to learn. His learning began at his conception and should continue to grow in unison with his body throughout his natural life. All learning takes place in the brain, but it is the body which acts as the vehicle by which knowledge is acquired. Both brain and body work together through the central nervous system (CNS), but both are dependent upon the senses for all information about the outer world.

When a child reaches school age it is generally assumed that the basic systems necessary for academic learning are established, and that good teaching, combined with the child's willingness to learn, will enable him to succeed. In order for him to be able to do this, at least three basic systems have to operate effectively:

Afferent system— information to the brain.

1. The reception of information via the senses.
2. The processing of information in the brain.
3. Response or expression to that information via the efferent system.

Efferent system— information from the brain to the body.

We have seen how the reflex system can affect performance at the levels of processing and response, causing brain stem reactions to direct the response without higher brain level involvement. Equally, distorted sensory input may awaken anew reflex activity which would otherwise be inhibited, and thus a vicious circle of distorted sensation and inappropriate response is established.

Hyper — oversensitive, inadequate filtering of extraneous sensation

It has long been accepted that defects in vision and in hearing will impede the learning process, but they are generally investigated in isolation by an expert in each field. Frequently the child is only examined for deficit in one area and further investigations into what a child sees, what he hears or how he experiences touch, are not carried out. **Visual and auditory hypersensitivity are just as much of a handicap to learning as loss in these areas, and in some cases both hyper and hypo can coexist in a child.** (Delacato 1974) Both vision and hearing are dependent upon the vestibular apparatus for their functioning, but the occupational therapist and the audiologist work in separate departments and may never know that they both see the same child—one whose main problem is located in the inner ear.

Hypo — undersensitive, inadequate sensations received

White sound— continuous background sensation, which is always present and intrudes upon other sensations.

When the system is overloaded, the child can go into a "shock" reaction. i.e. the sympathetic nervous system shuts down all sensation and ceases to respond to the stimulus. This may be interpreted as being under-sensitive, when in fact it is an extreme reaction to being oversensitive.

The sympathetic nervous system consists of a network of nerve fibers which—under stress ready the body for either flight or standing to fight. It does so by increasing the heartbeat, quickening breathing and enhancing the supply of oxygen to the muscles by siphoning the blood supply from the skin to the deep muscles.

Hence the pallor or the redness of the skin is a clue to the condition of the child.

The parasympathetic nervous system—its opposite partner in the balancing, self-regulating autonomic nervous system— increases salivary gland secretions, decreases the heart rate, promotes digestion and dilates the blood vessels.

None of the senses develop or operate in isolation. Each one is reinforced, modified and influenced by information from the others. Our language and our interpretation accepts cross-sensory reference as being fundamental to our understanding of the world: Hearing has been described as a "specialized sense of touch," we "taste with our nose," "feast with our eyes," "see with our fingers" and according to Tomatis we "read with our ears." We accept balance between the different aspects of our lives as being fundamental to health and to well-being, and yet "the sense of balance" is perhaps the forgotten sixth sense of the twentieth century. An understanding of the senses and how they complement one another is essential, if we are to understand and to help the child who cannot "make sense" of the world and therefore has difficulty learning through the accepted channels of education.

1. BALANCE AND THE VESTIBULAR SYSTEM

Balance is the core of functioning. It is the first system to be fully developed, becoming operational at 16 weeks in utero and is myelinated at birth, providing the fetus with a sense of direction and orientation inside the womb. It is in place to help cope with the problem of gravity, which the child will encounter in its full force for the first time when he is born.

The balance mechanism monitors all sensation in both directions between the brain and the body.

Every living creature shares one relationship: a relationship with gravity. It is gravity that provides us with our center, whether it be in space, in time, motion, depth or sense of self, acting as the nucleus from which all operations become possible. Problems in the balance system will have repercussions for all other areas of functioning. Such problems affect the sensory systems, because all sensation passes through the vestibular mechanism at brainstem level before being transmitted elsewhere for analysis.

The vestibular system operates closely with the reflexes to facilitate balance. It is located in the inner ear, and its job is to monitor and make adjustments to any movement of the head or the environment. *"As we move and interact with gravity, sensory receptors in the ear are activated, and impulses appraising the central nervous system about the position of the head in space are directed to various parts of the brain and down the spinal cord. It is believed that sensory impulses from the eyes, ears, muscles and joints must be matched to the vestibular input before such information can be reprocessed efficiently. If that is true, what we see, hear and feel makes sense only if the vestibular system is functioning adequately."* (Pyfer, J. & Johnson, R. 1981)

The Vestibular System has two main parts:

1.   Three fluid filled semicircular canals, set at right angles to each other.

2.   Two vestibular sacs, also filled with fluid.

Hair cells line the inside of both organs. Any movement of the body, particularly the head, sets up motion of the fluid in the canals and the sacs, stimulating the hair cells. Movement of the hair cells triggers the release of nerve signals which provide the brain with information about direction, angle and extent of the movement, so that appropriate muscle adjustments may be made. Certain hair cells are particularly sensitive to gravity, informing the brain of any deviation from the upright position. Signals from the vestibular system then pass along the vestibular nerve to the cerebellum. The cerebellum has been called "the moderator between sensation and brain level response" (Levinson 1981), as it coordinates information from the inner ear with other parts of the body. It monitors where we are in space and what position we are in, i.e. standing, sitting, running, climbing, somersaulting, etc. If information from the vestibular system is out of alignment with information from the other senses, motion sickness results. Astronauts experience a unique form of this when placed in a gravity-free environment where their sense of "center" is lost, and they rely heavily on tactile and visual stimuli to retain a sense of location.

It has long been recognized that sensory deprivation will result in emotional and physical distress. In extreme cases it has been used as a method of interrogation and torture resulting in irreversible insanity within a very short period of time. The unfortunate victim was blindfolded, placed in a suit which covered him from head to toe (depriving him of external tactile stimuli) and "white sound" was played into the ears through a headset. If this did not yield results, the victim was then placed in a centrifuge and spun for several minutes with devastating effect. Very few victims ever recovered their sanity.

The vestibular is possibly the oldest and the most primitive of the sensory systems. It is believed that the human ear is an outgrowth or development of one of the earliest vertebrate complex sensory end-organs—the lateral line receptor. The lateral line receptor probably had

Lateral line receptor: A sensory system found in many kinds of fish and some amphibians that informs the animal of water motion in relation to body surface.

57

its beginning in the armored fish of the Silurian period over 400 million years ago. Movement of the hairs situated in the sensitive areas of the lateral line receptor are used by fish to detect chemicals and electrical fields in surrounding water and thereby alert them to approaching obstacles, food and predators. [Note 1]

In mammals the ear has become more highly developed, dividing into two structures:
1.   The *vestibular* apparatus or *balance* mechanism.
2.   The *cochlea* or *auditory* apparatus.

Although they are often viewed as separate systems by specialists, they share a common chamber, fluid (endolymph) and transmission of information via the same cranial nerve, the VIIIth cranial nerve or vestibulo-acoustic nerve. Thus, hearing is bound to be influenced by information passing through the vestibular, and the vestibular is bound to be influenced by sound.

The relationship between the visual and vestibular systems is experienced in many ways.
For example, if the vestibular system is stimulated as a result of rotation or rocking, the sensation of "dizziness" gives the temporary illusion that the visual world is moving. If you are seated in a waiting train at a railway station and the train alongside you starts to move away, the vestibular system is fooled into thinking that the body is moving.

Both portions of the labyrinth are involved in the perception of motion, Madaule (1993) stated that it is the vestibular portion alone which monitors slow movement, but we also use the auditory component to judge the direction (orientation) speed and timing of any movement which travels faster than a speed of 20hz, by calculating the speed and distance between the two ears to locate where movement has occurred.

Steinbach (1994) suggests that "sound is not sound" but is the physical expression of movement or vibration. The ear then acts as a receptor and transmitter of vibration to be interpreted by the brain. Defects in the vestibular apparatus may affect the point at which the auditory system takes over, and problems in the auditory apparatus may result in the vestibular system working overtime to compensate.

Both the vestibular system and the reflex system are closely aligned to the visual system, acting as the substrata upon which oculo-motor and visual-perceptual skills are built. Impulses from the vestibular system to the brainstem affect equilibrium reactions, with motor nerves that control eye-movements and with nerves that lead to the somatosensory portion of the cerebral cortex. [Note 2]

Signals to and from the vestibular system in the inner ear pass through four nuclei —the vestibular nuclei— in the pons of the brainstem.[Note 7] The vestibular nuclei serve as a junction for messages passing between the balance mechanism and the body via the Vestibular Spinal System, and for signals passing between the balance mechanism and the eyes along the Vestibular Ocular Reflex Arc (VOR). A further connection links both systems to the cerebellum, whose task is to modulate and regulate communication and output from all of these centers so that movement is smooth and controlled. [Notes 3, 4, 5]

The vestibular and reflex systems are inter-dependent in the control of posture and movement. Vestibular dysfunction can alter the level of reflex response, and reflex abnormalities can impede the functioning of the vestibular system.

The vestibular system has connections to:
- The autonomic nervous system — digestion, etc.
- The visual system — 90% of cells in the visual system respond to vestibular stimulation.
- The sleep and waking cycles
- REM dream sleep
- The perception of weight

(King L.J., Schrager O.L. 1999)

"Vestibular input is necessary for static and dynamic balance development, eye-tracking ability and motor planning. Children who are slow to develop good vestibular functioning are delayed in all gross motor patterns which require coordination of both sides of the body. They may have difficulty in maintaining posture, with eye-hand coordination, and with fine motor control." (Pyfer 1981)

Inappropriate vestibular signals may elicit primitive reflex reactions, but equally, aberrant reflex activity will impede the activities of the vestibular system. If a child is to utilize the information provided for him by his senses, there must be a balance between them.

****

Signs suggestive of vestibular dysfunction:

— **Poor balance**
— **Delay in postural and motor milestones such as head control, sitting, crawling and walking**
— **Poor muscle tone**
— **Motion sickness beyond the age of puberty**
— **Dislike of heights, swings, carousels, escalators and lifts, or conversely, no fear of heights**
— **Easily disoriented, poor sense of direction**
— **Clumsy**
— **Difficulty remaining still; may actively seek vestibular stimulation through activities such as excessive rocking or spinning**
— **Difficulties in space perception**
— **Poor organizational skills, "dizzy" or scatterbrained behavior**
— **Cannot work out "how" to do certain activities, eg. push/pull**
— **Fatigue/lethargy**
— **Inability to mentally rotate or reverse objects in space or procedures; can affect such things as the ability to read an analog clock which is a spatial ability, or to understand that multiplication and division are the same processes in reverse**

****

TACTILITY

Although the vestibular system is the first to be fully developed and myelinated, it is the sense of touch which provides us with our first source of contact with the outer world. The first observed response to tactile stimulation occurs at approximately five weeks after conception with the emergence of the mass cutaneous withdrawal reflexes mentioned in Chapter 1. Gentle stimulation of the upper lip results in immediate withdrawal from the source of contact by the whole organism. The area of sensitivity rapidly spreads over the next four weeks to encompass the oral region of the face, the palms of the hands and the soles of the feet, until eventually the whole body surface is responsive to touch. However, the earliest primitive realization of touch is a defensive one characterized by withdrawal.

During the second and third trimesters of pregnancy tactile awareness should mature to allow the grasping reflexes to develop (palmar, plantar, rooting, suck, Moro, etc.), so that by the time the baby is born, touch is associated with security, with feeding, comfort and eventually exploration. Touch precedes both hearing and vision as the primary channel of learning: Touch receptors cover the entire body.

The area in the brain which perceives touch stretches like a headband and is called the somatosensory cortex. It is capable of registering heat, cold, pressure, pain and body position. The most sensitive areas of the body have a correspondingly large representation area in the somato-sensory cortex, with the lips, hands and genital regions occupying a large section of the somatosensory map. Even the base of the hair follicles have touch receptors. The vestibular apparatus functions through the movement of fluid over hair cells, the sense of touch is essential for the functioning of balance, orientation and motion.

Ayres (1980) divided the tactile system into protective and discrimin-ative subsystems: Protective receptors are located around the hair follicles and respond to subtle stimulation such as sound and air waves (vibration) moving across the body. *"They literally tell us where our body ends and where space begins."* (Pyfer 1981).

Discriminative receptors are located in the dermis and respond when we come into contact with something—either actively or passively. These systems should be mutually exclusive, that is: one shuts down as the other comes into action. The protective system stays in operation until we are touched, and unless that contact is threatening, the discriminative system comes into play as soon as contact takes place.

Dermis—
top layer of the skin.

The child who has an over-active protective system will be "tactile defensive" and may still have uninhibited cutaneous withdrawal reflexes which continue to influence the central nervous system. If this is the case, then touch can be neither an instant source of comfort nor a purveyor of information, for the reflex response will elicit withdrawal from the source of contact, and the child cannot adequately utilize his tactile discrimination skills. The "hyper-tactile" child may have abnormal perception in all input to the area of the cortex which registers touch. He may have poor tolerance and/or adaptive mechanisms to heat and cold. He may have a low pain threshold, particularly to pain associated with piercing the skin, but, paradoxically, a high tolerance to internal pain.

This may be the child who over-reacts to injections, grazes and small cuts, but who will fail to notice that his legs are covered with bruises. He may dislike any form of physical contact and therefore have difficulty in either receiving or demonstrating affection, which makes it difficult for the mother to establish a warm relationship with the child. He may appear to be inordinately stubborn about the clothes he wears and the way that he does things. Contact sports may be avoided, and the child may have a poor body image and sense of his own space.

In extreme cases, this may play a significant part in the distortion of body image, which is characteristic of anorexia nervosa. The anorexic "feels" herself to be fat and believes her own body space to occupy a far greater area than it actually does. Despite all attempts to shrink from within, no amount of weight loss will alter this sensation, as proportionally the same amount of skin surface and therefore number of receptors remain in contact with the outer world. Because sensation of this type is mediated at the brainstem, the feeling will over-ride any logic that is imposed from the cortex, and no amount of evidence to the contrary will change the anorexic's perception of herself.

Tactile discrimination should provide us with an enormous amount of information about our environment. Studies with rats have shown that offspring handled in the laboratory have better immune systems and gain weight better. Early handling also leads to permanent sensitivity of the part of the brain that controls the stress response, resulting in reduced levels of stress hormones. Without touch, small children rapidly become disturbed and may attempt to supply themselves with essential sensory information by self-stimulation. One example of this is the institutionalized "rocking" observed amongst so many children abandoned in orphanages. Too often it is assumed to be a sign of mental retardation instead of being regarded as an attempt by the child to provide himself with essential vestibular, tactile and proprioceptive information. Studies of premature infants have shown a 45% increase in weight gain amongst children who are massaged for 15 minutes, three times a day. [Note 6]

Touch is important for a child to develop his/her body image— sometimes referred to as a mental picture or map of the body. Many children with Dyspraxia have a poor sense of body image, difficulty locating different parts of their body in space and have inadequate awareness of whole sections of their own bodies. When drawing a picture of a human figure, often the head is drawn disproportionately large with little or no neck (often a feature of drawings of children who have underdeveloped headrighting reflexes). Drawings of large hands and "awkward" limbs or stance are also indications of problems.

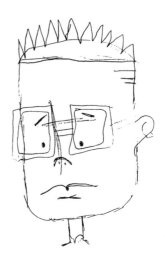

This figure is eight year old boy's drawing of a human figure before starting a reflex stimulation/inhibition program.

This boy had a diagnosis of severe Dyslexia and his teacher had suggested to his mother he also seemed to demonstrate features of Asperger's Syndrome. Note the large head (he had an unusually large head) and the fact that he makes no attempt to draw a body.

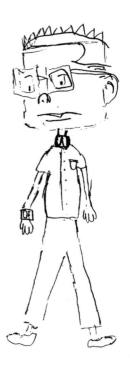

Drawing of a human figure after nine months on a reflex stimulation/inhibition program.

Although the head is still drawn disporportionately large, the rest of the body is now also drawn.

One of the tests for soft signs of neurological dysfunction is the Tandem Walk. The children are asked to walk forward, slowly placing one foot in front of another with the heel touching the toe of the other. Children with reflex problems can't locate their feet without looking at them, or else they leave large spaces between each foot. Such signs indicate that they have poor proprioceptive awareness of where different parts of their body are in space without reinforcement from the visual system.

One nine year old child, who had been adopted from one of the former Eastern Bloc countries at the age of three and a half, who had spent the first three years of her life confined to a cot with no opportunity for gross movement, always drew herself without legs. After several months on a reflex stimulation/inhibition program which involved carrying out exercises lying on the back and moving her legs through space with her eyes closed, her "self-portraits" included her legs.

In the early months of life, it is the mouth—through rooting, sucking and exploring with the lips and tongue—which provides the neonate and the infant with its primary source of tactile information. The hands are also involved —initially in palmar movements and Babkin response— and then later, in an interplay between hand and mouth. This is the so-called "oral" phase of development. As in the growth of prenatal tactile response, postnatal tactile development starts with the mouth and spreads outward to the hands, the feet and eventually the entire body. If either tactile withdrawal or grasp reflexes remain prevalent beyond their allotted time, they will disrupt the delicate balance between the protective and the discriminative tactile systems.

Babkin response during nursing: palming movements in the hands causing pursing of the lips. Sucking movements may result in kneading motions of the hands —kittens also do this when being fed.

As children grow older, physical contact with the parents diminishes. At puberty the adolescent tentatively seeks tactile stimulation anew with the blossoming of sexual awareness, so that a cycle of search for contact continues through life. It is perhaps the 8-16 year old age group who will suffer most if they have undetected tactile problems, for this is the age when the child must seek tactile information for himself— parents and teachers no longer supply it with the richness that they did during infancy. The child who lacks sufficient protective control will be the dare-devil, who does not sense danger, is frequently oblivious to injury either to himself or to others, and who cannot read other people's body language. He presents a danger to himself and everyone around him—he is literally "thick-skinned," unlike his tactile defensive counterpart who will shy away from activities and experiences for which he is inadequately equipped.

****

Symptoms of hypertactility.

1 **Hypersensitivity**
2. **Dislike of being touched, but may be a compulsive "toucher"**
3. **Allergic skin reactions**
4. **Poor temperature control**
5. **Low external pain threshold**
6. **Anorexia**
7. **Dislike of sports**
8. **Tendency to rely on sensory instead of verbal language**

****

Symptoms of hypotactility.

1. **Hypotactile**
2. **High threshold of pain**
3. **Craving for contact sports**
4. **Child may provoke roughhousing or fighting**
5. **Compulsive touching**
6. **"Bull in a china shop"**

AUDITORY

Hearing, like vestibular sensation and touch, is the reception and transmission of energy through motion and vibration. The human ear is a compound development, forming during the second half of the embryonic period (4-8 weeks in utero). As the ossicles of the middle ear develop, central nervous system connections are established to the cochlea and the vestibular structures. Myelination of auditory fibers occurs between the 24th and the 28th week in utero, and sound perception develops slowly from this time onward. At this stage, the ear is tuned specifically to the sounds heard in utero, but the fetus will respond to some external auditory stimuli as well.

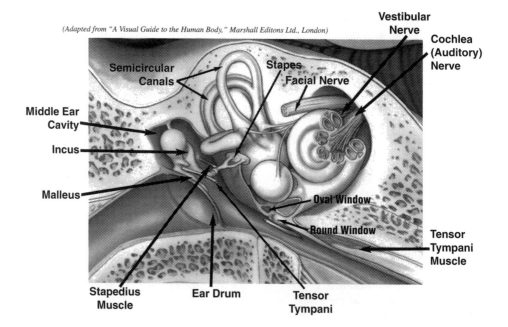

(Adapted from "A Visual Guide to the Human Body," Marshall Editons Ltd., London)

For the first few days after birth the ears are still filled with superfluous fluid (similar to the water in the ears after swimming or bathing), with the result that the infant inhabits an auditory no-man's-land between uterine and extra-uterine sound. Once the fluid has cleared, the neonate ears become receptive to a vast range of sound frequencies, something in the region of 0-20,000 Hertz and beyond.

The number of vibrations will determine the pitch of the sound heard. e.g. 125 Hz is low sound, 8000 Hz is perceived as high sound.

During the first three years of life, the child must learn to use his ears to "tune-in" to the specific frequencies of his own language, in much the same way that a radio is adjusted to select specific stations. It is at this time that the child has the potential to learn any language if it is exposed to the sounds of that language continuously over a period of time, no matter what language his mother speaks. After the age of three years, when these fine tuning adjustments should have been made, it becomes far more difficult to assimilate a new language.

Hearing **loss** has long been recognized as being an enormous handicap linguistically, educationally and socially. Much less attention has been paid until recently to problems of hearing **discrimination** amongst children with learning difficulties or with language disorders. Speech may have developed at the correct time, but the more detailed analysis of sounds essential for reading and spelling may have been omitted: The child cannot hear the difference between similar or blended sounds such as "ch" and "sh," "th" and "f," "p" and "b." If the letters sound the same to him, he presumes that they should be spelled the same way. Storr (1993) discusses two essential components for reading—vision and hearing. He talks about the "auditory reader" who is not just a phonetic reader, but who reads silently with an "inner voice" which enables him to see and hear the words inside his head, as if they were being read out loud. Poor auditory discrimination skills will impede this process.

Frequent ear, nose and throat infections in early childhood resulting in intermittent hearing loss over a period of time can prevent the development of such auditory discrimination skills. Lack of auditory stimulation, or even a constant cacophony of background noise in early life can discourage early "listening" and the child may learn to shut out and ignore sound from an early age.

TECTORIAL MEMBRANE   HAIR BUNDLES

HAIR CELLS

BASILAR MEMBRANE

AUDITORY NERVE

Hair cells responding to sound
Adapted from George Von Békésy, 1957

Scientists in New York using a superconducting quantum interference device (SQID), which senses tiny changes in magnetic fields on a brain listening to music, have found an eerie reflection of the black and white keys of a piano responding in the brain to the notes that were heard. *"The brain hears loud sounds in a totally different place from quieter sounds, but the areas which register tones are laid out like a keyboard."* (Williamson 1992). It is possible that failure to register specific sounds at the crucial stage for language learning may result in part of the keyboard or sound map being omitted or ceasing to respond.

Hearing too much or "auditory hypersensitivity" can be just as much of a problem as hearing deficit. The inability to filter or occlude miscellaneous sound, suggests poorly developed listening skills, and can have profound effect upon later learning, language, communication, and behavior. In the last 20 years research has turned to focus upon the problems of "listening," as opposed to problems of hearing. Tomatis, in France, and Christian Volf, in Denmark, quite independently of each other, were pioneers in this approach. Since then, various techniques have been devised to assess and to retrain the listening skills of individuals with such diverse problems as autism, hyperactivity, dyslexia, depression and imperfect pitch discrimination amongst musicians.

Some children who are initially either <u>left</u> ear preferred or who show <u>no</u> clear ear preference when first tested using binaural stimulation and dichotic listening tests, become <u>more</u> left-eared for a short period of time when they start on auditory discrimination training, suggesting that it may be developmentally normal to be left-eared at certain stages of language acquisition, and that right-ear preference is an indication of maturity in language development. This would fit with Allan Schore's theory of continuous interchange between the left and right hemispheres of the cortex during the learning stages of new skills.

Tomatis has shown that there is a difference in the way that sounds are transmitted to the language processing center in the brain, depending on which ear is used as the dominant listening ear. The <u>right</u> ear is the most efficient of the two for receiving and transmitting sounds of language, and left-eared children may be at a disadvantage. Sounds heard through the right ear pass directly to the main language center in the left hemisphere (Fig.A). Sounds heard via the <u>left</u> ear pass first to the sub-language center in the right hemisphere and then have to pass through the corpus callosum to the left hemisphere for decoding (Fig.B). There is a delay in milliseconds, similar to the delay experienced on an overseas telephone call, while the sounds pass to the satellite and down again. The child who is primarily left-eared may have difficulty in following a list of verbal instructions as he is still decoding the first two instructions when the third is being given. The child who suffers from auditory delay may also appear to be slow or slightly "vacant" when spoken to.

Fig. A   Fig. B

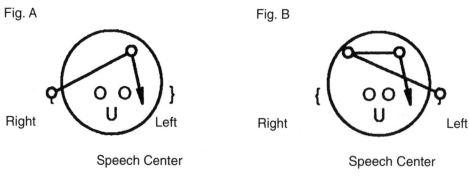

Right   Left   Right   Left

Speech Center   Speech Center

<u>Lack</u> of ear preference may further confuse the situation, resulting in sounds reaching the brain in a different order from the order they are

arranged phonetically in a word, i.e. the child who switches ear preference while listening or sounding out a word may find the sounds processed through the <u>left</u> ear arrive a fraction later than the sounds processed through the <u>right</u> ear, irrespective of their correct order. For example, if the word phon/et/ic was heard, using the <u>left</u> ear for the first syllable and the <u>right</u> ear for the latter two, it may arrive at the brain as "eticphon" or even "etphonic." Inconsistencies in spelling involving letter, syllable and word reversals are a logical outcome.

If the child is to be able to hear words and then to separate specific sounds and distinguish the phonemes and formants in them, he needs to have excellent hearing throughout the range of frequencies from 125 Hz to 8000 Hz. Every language has its unique frequency band, within which fall all the sounds used in that language. Key stages or windows for learning are well known, and if that key stage is missed, the chances of subsequently developing skills in that area are considerably reduced. The "window" for language is during the first three years of life—exactly the same time that the ears should be making their fine tuning adjustments. The child learns to filter out unnecessary sounds, and tune in to the sounds of language, so that he can start to hear and to reproduce the sounds necessary for speech and later for written language.

dB — decibels: measure of volume of sound

A volume of 20dB is considered normal. A volume of 40dB would be considered adequate but not ideal for a child to cope in a noisy classroom by most school doctors or audiologists whose primary job is to detect hearing deficit. Thus, a child whose hearing falls between 20 and 40dB will not be considered sufficiently at-risk to warrant treatment. Nevertheless, this type of hearing can have a profound effect upon the child's ability to discriminate between similar but different sounds such as "sh" and "ch," "f" and "th," etc. We should consider 40-60dB moderate hearing loss; 60dB and beyond, severe hearing loss.

20dB is approximately the volume of a quiet telephone conversation

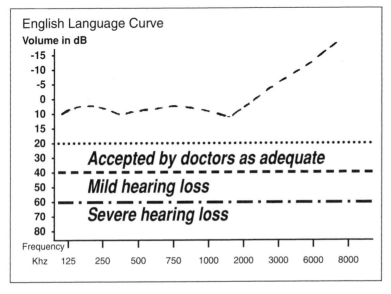

English Language Curve

As the chart on the previous page demonstrates, however, the English language curve requires discrimination at levels far more sensitive than 20dB, particularly in the high frequencies which are involved in sounds such as f, s, sh, ch, th, etc. Vowel and consonant sounds cross the spectrum of frequencies so that minor deviations from the language curve may cause specific speech and spelling problems.

The difference between b and d, p and q, is one of directionality, but the decision as to which way the symbol should face is based upon the fact that each letter *sounds* different. If a child has difficulty in distinguishing a difference between the *sound* of these letters (b and p are close to each other in terms of frequency and both are sounds which it is difficult to tell apart on the lips), the rationale for writing each letter one way or the other is meaningless. Similarly, f, th, sh, ch sounds in the English language are hard to distinguish if there is any high frequency hearing loss, and these are letters and blends which are often incorrectly used by children with spelling difficulties and Dyslexia.

Some children suffer from hyperacuity, but as this is not measured in standard hearing tests, the child is again dismissed as not having a problem. Hearing too much can result in enormous concentration difficulties, speech difficulties and problems with social interaction. Tomatis described how high frequency sound is "energizing" while low frequency sound tends to be relaxing or "enervating." Clinical tests on a number of hyperactive children at The Institute for Neuro-Physiological Psychology have revealed them to be hypersensitive in the <u>high</u> frequency range of sounds, in some cases still perceiving sounds between 2000 and 6000 Hz at a volume of (minus) -10 dB and below. One boy was even convinced he had extra-sensory perception as he knew a car was coming round a corner several seconds before anyone else. He was very upset when it was suggested to him that he did have "super" sensory perception, but only because his hearing was so acute!

Dr. Kjeld Johansen, at the Dyslexia Research Laboratory in Gudhjem, Denmark, has devised a system of assessing and treating problems of auditory discrimination and auditory processing. Over 20 years of independent research developed from the original ideas of Christian Volf have resulted in a therapeutic approach which has been statistically proven to be effective. Audiometric tests are carried out to measure monaural thresholds and to determine hearing acuity throughout the hearing range. A dichotic listening test is also used to establish which is the primary leading ear. Once the tests have been analyzed, children are given an audio tape to listen to for 10 minutes per day. Specific tapes have been made in which all sounds except the frequencies they have difficulty hearing have been filtered out. By listening to pure frequencies unpolluted by extraneous sound, children can start to "hear" the sounds that they were formerly unable to discriminate. The tapes are also specially adjusted to encourage right eared listening. The tapes are altered at 6-8 weekly intervals, and hearing rechecked every few months to insure that improvements are occurring. As the children's listening skills improve, concomitant changes take place in reading, writing, use of language and behavior.

The value of music for learning has long been recognized, but with financial cut backs and changes in methods of education, music has taken a back seat in the early learning years of many children. Vast improvements have been made in electronic sound equipment. Because it is so inexpensive and easily available, a lot of music is now heard through tapes, discs or synthesizers where many of the beneficial high frequency sounds are lost.

Live music—sadly—is today a rare experience for many children. Previous generations of children learned multiplication tables, alphabet and Latin verbs to tunes. Understanding of what they had learned came later, but the tune and the rhythm aided recall. Most people can still remember the words to all the verses of any hymn if someone sings the first few notes of the tune for them. Without the music, they cannot find the words. The Master of Choristers at an English cathedral said that the reading age of all his choir boys improved by 12 months within 6 months of their joining the choir. This remained true irrespective of whether they were good or poor readers at the time of joining. It could be said that this was the direct result of the amount of written material they had to sing, but it could also be said that the dual processes of listening, vocalizing, and learning to hear pitch and rhythm enhanced other skills. Dr. Audrey Wisbey, in Cambridge, found much the same reading improvement. Cathedrals and other large old public buildings have acoustics which are rich in the high frequencies, which are lost in the low ceiling, carpeted and cushioned buildings of our time.

"Sound is not sound." (Steinbach 1994) Sound is vibration, motion and energy. If we hear no sound we perceive danger, for the totally silent world is a dead world. Sound passes through all levels of the brain, affecting not just the ear and the vestibular but also our bodies through bone conduction. The significance of sound for learning is immeasurable.

****
Symptoms of auditory problems.
1. **Short attention span**
2. **Distractibility**
3. **Hypersensitivity to sounds**
4. **Misinterpretation of questions**
5. **Confusion of similar sounding words, frequent need to have a word repeated**
6. **Inability to follow sequential instructions**
7. **Flat and monotonous voice**
8. **Hesitant speech**
9. **Weak vocabulary**
10. **Poor sentence structure**
11. **Inability to sing in tune**
12. **Confusion or reversal of letters**
13. **Poor reading comprehension**
14. **Poor reading aloud**
15. **Poor spelling**
16. **Auditory delay**
****

VISUAL

Vision is obviously essential for academic learning. The skills of reading, writing, spelling and arithmetic are all dependent upon the ability to see written symbols. When learning difficulties arise, vision is often the first area to be checked. If the child passes a simple eye test which only assesses distance vision, further investigation into visual problems are seldom pursued. Distance vision is only one component in the complex sense of sight. How we see, the way that we use our eyes and how we perceive the world through sight, is the result of a complex series of connections and neural developments which should have taken place in the early formative years, and which are dependent upon adequate maturation of the central nervous system. (CNS)

Oculomotor, visual-perceptual and visual-motor integration skills are just as vital for learning as is good distance vision.

X

Left eye   Right eye

Each eye sees a different image; the brain must fuse the two. First of all, both eyes must work as a team, so that each eye is directed to the same fixation point on the page, rather like two spotlights highlighting a dancer on the center of the stage. This is called convergence and must be fully developed for the child to perceive one clear picture. Operating as a team, the eyes should scan along a line of letters and send a clear image to the brain. The next figure shows the drawings of one 13 year old boy whose eyes never learned to converge, so that he still sees two separate images on the paper. It is not surprising that he has enormous difficulties with all written material.

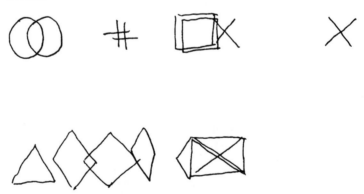

Figure A on the next page shows the drawing by a boy whose eyes were not working together as a team when he was first assessed. It was his first attempt at copying a picture of a Jaguar sports car—a meaningless jumble of scribbles. Sometime later, the Child Psychologist who had assessed him asked him to attempt the drawing again, but this time with one eye covered. Figure B was the result.

When asked why he had drawn it so differently, the boy's comment was "I thought that everybody else saw flat images like my first drawing and could somehow turn it into the second." Because the two eyes were not functioning as a team (yoking), the image he was seeing was fragmented and unstable. By removing the confusion of the second image, he was able to make sense of the material in front of him and reproduce it remarkably well. This is not a case for eye patching as a solution to the problem because the two eyes have to learn to work *together*. Eye patching does not develop yoking ability, but this example demonstrates the devastating effect of a combination of convergence difficulties and lack of yoking ability upon visual functioning.

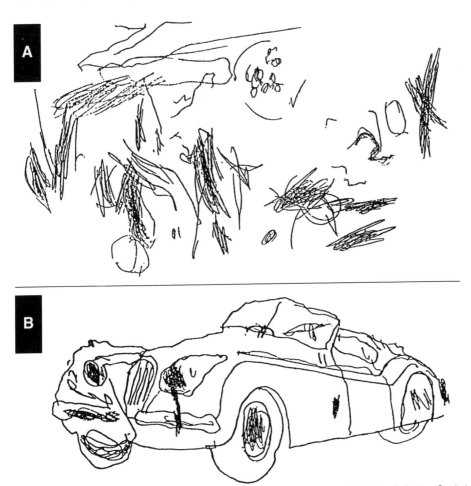

(Printed by permission of Catharina Johannesson Alvegard, The Institute for Neuro-Physiological Psychology. Gothenberg, Sweden)

A second necessity is that the image seen by each eye must be sharp—clearly focused. The focus must be adjusted quickly from one distance or one angle to another. This skill is called <u>accommodation</u>. Difficulties with either accommodation or convergence can affect one another.

After that, in order to read easily, it is necessary to be able to scan or track along a line of print smoothly and evenly, so that the brain can receive a flow of sequentially correct information. Tracking is vital for orderly progression from one word to another, or finding the way from line to line without loss of place. In addition to the three skills of convergence, accommodation and tracking, a child also needs to have good directional awareness to distinguish similar but directionally different symbols such as p/q, b/d, on/no, left/felt, etc. (Duighan 1994)

> *Directional awareness is a vestibular based skill. The vestibular system acts like an internal compass to give us a sense of "center" from which we can automatically judge up from down, left from right, start from finish. The development of cerebral dominance at the age of 7-8 years cements this knowledge, but the problems with direction may still persist after cerebral dominance has occurred if vestibular functioning is faulty. This may be the child who gets easily lost in new surroundings, has difficulty learning to tell time on an old fashioned clock and who has poor organizational skills.*

Reading difficulty is only the tip of the iceberg where visual problems are concerned. Handwriting and spelling will also be profoundly affected, as is coordination, because the child will have poor spatial awareness, poor body image and impaired hand-eye coordination. Many sports and leisure activities will only be performed with great effort, and levels of attainment will be disproportionate to the energy and enthusiasm initially applied to the task. The child will become frustrated, and may soon start to avoid activities enjoyed by other children and thus unwittingly increase his own sense of isolation. It has been suggested (Trevor-Roper 1990) that visual difficulties directly influence the choice of subjects, hobbies and eventually the career that an individual will make.

Myopic — short sighted: good near-distance vision, poor distance vision beyond 12 to 24 inches.

Trevor-Roper cites the myopic child as the child who rarely becomes a good sportsman, and who concentrates upon artistic or "bookish" pastimes, which fall directly within his field of nearpoint vision. He links developments in the Impressionist school of painting to the corresponding deterioration in the artists' eyesight during the later years of their lives, when clarity of form in their paintings increasingly gave way to the representation of the interplay of light forms.

Since poor visual information will impair the recognition and recall of groups of letters either as units or as a picture (visio-spatial awareness), spelling will be affected. Visual imagery or visualization is necessary for spelling, as it enables the child to form templates or a visual memory for words in the mind's eye. These are then matched against the written word to assess whether the word "looks" right, i.e. is there a variable within the word which does not correspond to the remembered visual image of that word? As our hearing deteriorates gradually over the years, we use auditory memory to continue to speak and to pronounce words correctly. So, also do we need a visual memory to be able to write and to spell words accurately.

The effect of aberrant reflex activity upon oculomotor functioning was discussed in Chapter 1, with the asymmetrical tonic neck reflex

(ATNR) having an adverse effect upon tracking, the tonic labyrinthine reflex (TLR) upon convergence, the Moro reflex upon fixation and the symmetrical tonic neck reflex STNR upon the readjustment of binocular vision from one distance to another.

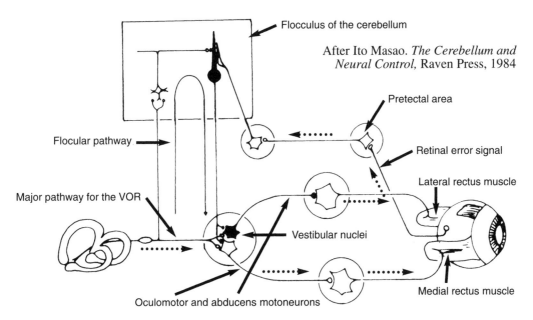

After Ito Masao. *The Cerebellum and Neural Control,* Raven Press, 1984

Dysfunction in these areas will inevitably result in visual-perceptual difficulties. It is important that an examination be carried out to assess what a child sees and to investigate the way his eyes work together. On the next page are two examples of severe visual-perceptual difficulties. Both children were in a normal school struggling to keep up with academic work. They were asked to copy the Tansley Standard Figures and the Bender Visual Gestalt Figures.

Despite a history of reading, writing and spelling difficulties, the visual-perceptual and visual-motor integration skills of these children had not previously been investigated. Child A and Child B also had a cluster of aberrant primitive reflexes.

It must be remembered that the eye is only an instrument of vision. To make effective use of the sights eyes provide, the child must also make use of other sensory information. The foundations for these inter-connections are laid down during the first year of life, at the time that neural pathways are formed between the eye, the brain and the body. Vision is particularly dependent upon one of these pathways: the Vestibulo Ocular Reflex Arc (VOR).

Interaction between the components of this loop will determine the efficiency of the visual system in later life: i.e. the rapid exchange of information between the vestibular apparatus, the eyes, and the level of reflex response to incoming stimuli. Any defect in one of these elements will affect the smooth operation of the whole.

Bender-Gestalt test

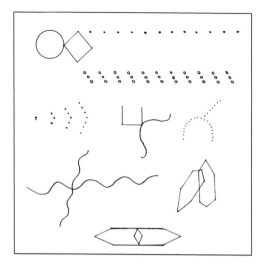

Child A — First test on left, second test after 5 months therapy on right

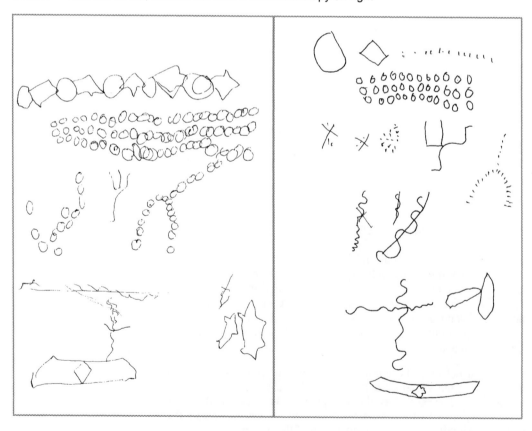

Tansley Standard Visual Figures test

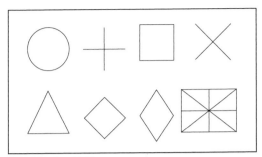

A.E. Tansley 1967

Child B — First test (top figure), second test (bottom figure) after 3 months therapy.

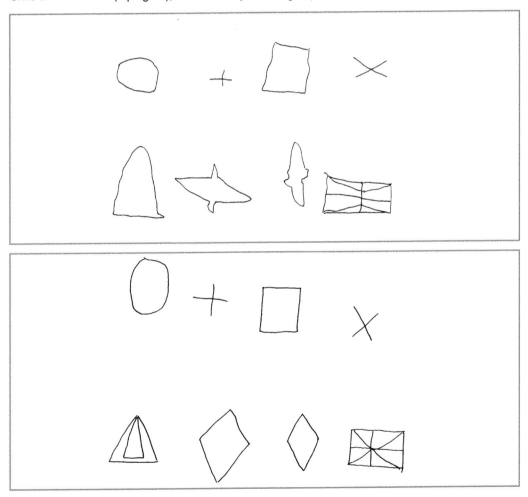

****

Symptoms indicative of visual stress:

1. Misreading words
2. Missing or repeating words or lines
3. Slow reading
4. Need to use finger or marker as a pointer
5. Inability to remember what has been read
6. Poor concentration
7. Child describes letters which "move," "jump" or are poorly focused
8. Reading at a very close distance
9. Reading with one eye covered or sideways posture
10. Distractibility (stimulus bound effect)
11. Poor posture when reading or writing
12. Poorly spaced work
13. Handwriting crooked, or slopes in different directions, letters poorly balanced
14. Clumsiness
15. Difficulty with ball games.
16. Headaches

****

PROPRIOCEPTION

Closely allied to the other senses and interdependent upon them is the compound sense of proprioception. While it is the result of multi-sensory information, it also forms an information channel of its own. Proprioception or kinesthesis enables us to know where parts of our body are at any time and to make the appropriate postural adjustments. It is an internal sense of physical self which allows us to carry out detailed maneuvers without conscious awareness and in the absence of other sensory cues.

Proprioceptors are located throughout the body in the joints, tendons, muscles, etc. Their input is processed primarily through the vestibular system, but also coordinates with information from all other sensory sources to influence body movements and direct adjustments for fine muscle coordination. Needless to say, distorted information coming from any one of these sources will also affect proprioception.

> *While proprioception and kinesthesis are often used interchangeably, the term proprioception encompasses all sensations involving body position, either at rest or in motion, the term kinesthesia refers only to sensations arising when active muscle contraction becomes involved. Thus, some children who have little proprioceptive input when they sit still, may constantly have to move because they rely on information from the muscle movement on where they are in space.*

> *In such a case, visual skills should also be checked.*

Poor proprioceptive awareness is common among children with learning difficulties. Paradoxically, a small number will rely too heavily upon either proprioception or kinesthesis to perform certain tasks. For example: A seven year old boy was asked to throw a bean bag into a box of sand from a distance of ten feet. The first four attempts missed the target, but on the fifth, the bag dropped into the box. Each subsequent throw was successful, until the box was moved one foot closer to him. Theoretically, this should have been easier, but he overshot the target at the next five throws. Thomas had poor depth perception and was relying upon proprioceptive information to direct the force of his throw. Once he had been successful he knew the "feel" of the throw necessary to hit the target. The same "feel" could not be useful to him once the target was moved.

Many children with poor individual sensory perception will attempt to use proprioception instead of the primary channel for learning. It is rather like using a huge net in an attempt to catch one individual fish. Learning can only be consistently successful if eyes, ears and balance system are also providing accurate information about changing circumstances. The child who attempts to use proprioception to compensate for weakness in another channel may be the child for whom "practice makes perfect . . . sometimes" and who will, at times, produce excellent results but appears to be inconsistent in his performance.

The child who will trace the shape of a letter or figure with his finger may be the one who cannot "see" it clearly. This may result in the development of splinter skills. The child will make the teacher believe he can do something, but she does not realize he has acquired a skill which cannot help him when it comes to more sophisticated learning.

****

Symptoms of poor proprioception

1. **Poor posture**
2. **Constant fidgeting or moving**
3. **Excessive desire to be held**
4. **May provoke fights to get sensory input**
5. **May have visual problems**
6. **Poorly developed knowledge of where different parts of the body are in space**

****

TASTE AND SMELL

The significance of taste and smell for learning is perhaps largely concentrated in the earliest years of a child's life, when his mouth is his primary source of information, exploration, expression and satisfaction. What does it taste like? Is it soft? Can I chew it? How big is it? etc. All early discoveries are made through the mouth.

Much of taste is dependent upon the sense of smell, as we know only too well when we have a bad cold and can only taste the specific tongue tastes of salty, bitter, sweet, and sour. Smell is, perhaps, the most evocative of all the senses, instantaneously spanning decades in its ability to remind us of a certain place, person or event. Instead of being routed through the thalamus—like the other sensory information —the nerves in the nasal passages send messages directly to the brain's olfactory bulbs which then spread the impulses to areas of the brain where memories are stored. Thus, a certain perfume will remind us of our mother when we were a small child and she was dressed up to go out for the evening, or the typical sounds and smells of a country we have visited. Smell can instantly summon multisensory images. It can also stimulate the production of hormones involved in the control of appetite, temperature and sexuality—the same region in the brain influenced by the Moro reflex: the hypothalamus.

The smell of school can easily become associated with stress, the smell of a hospital with pain.

Taste and smell provide important information about an ever changing environment. Their significance to learning is hard to pinpoint, but as they evoke memories of past experiences, they enrich a child's understanding of what the teacher is trying to convey.

****

Symptoms of Problems with Taste or Smell

HYPER
1. **Child may avoid going to the bathroom and is at risk of wetting his pants he because he cannot stand the smell of the antiseptics used**
2. **Child may avoid other children, especially those who come to school with dirty or smelly clothes**
3. **Child may misbehave after floors have been polished**
4. **Child may avoid eating in the cafeteria or be "faddy" about foods which have a strong smell**
5. **Dislike of close proximity to other people**

HYPO
   Child may eat indiscriminately, is at risk of eating substances labeled _Keep out of reach of children_.

****

SUMMARY

In some cases, sensory imbalance can be used to produce a rare streak of genius. For example, the accomplished musician who has highly sensitive and highly developed hearing in a specific range; the artist who is able to use slight visual distortion to create an image of the world that is truly unique; the writer, who is able to summon up emotion, experience and imaginations to give birth to a rich tapestry of characters and events; the actress who can literally feel herself into someone else's persona. These people have been able to gain insight from their particular sensory experience, and they have also had the skills which allowed them to turn this unusual ability to their advantage. The child who experiences failure from an early age on lacks the skill with which to profit from his own special window on the world. Our sensory receptors provide us with such an open window, through which we feel, perceive and maintain contact with the world around us.

Deprivation of even one of the senses will have a profound effect upon the individual, as will any alteration in the transmission of information via one of the sensory channels. Mode, intensity and duration of sensation are also of prime significance, as the type and degree of sensory input will directly influence the level of response that is given. Too little sensation may result in lack of response. Too much, may result in overreaction or vastly increased levels of stress as the individual attempts to maintain control over his response. Distortion or blurring of sensation may result in confusion and inappropriate response.

Finally, there needs to be a balance between the different sensory channels so that cross-sensory reference may occur, in order to provide the individual with multi-sensory information about his environment, to which he may then adapt his responses. This is sensory integration. When assessing a child with learning, language or behavioral difficulties, it is not sufficient to merely identify a hearing problem, a reading problem, a coordination problem, etc. It is necessary to look further and to ask, What does he hear? How does he see? Under which specific situations is his balance poor? Does he have the mature combination of movements necessary to read, to write and to speak? If a child does not see, hear or move in the way that it is assumed he should, the very foundations of learning are lacking.

Chapter 5

REFLEX TESTING

Tests listed:

1. Moro Reflex Standard Test
2. Moro Reflex Erect Test (Clarke, Bennett, and Rowston)
3. Palmar Reflex
4. Asymmetrical Tonic Neck Reflex Standard Test
5. Asymmetrical Tonic Neck Reflex Schilder Test
6. Rooting Reflex
7. Suck Reflex
8. Spinal Galant Reflex
9. Tonic Labyrinthine Reflex Erect Test
10. Symmetrical Tonic Neck Test
11. Landau Reflex
12. Amphibian Reflex Prone—Supine
13. Segmental Rolling Reflex Hips Shoulders
14. Oculo-Headrighting Reflexes
15. Labyrinthine Headrighting Reflexes

The following test procedures relating to reflexes discussed in the text should be used for purposes of identification only, as they represent just <u>one</u> <u>section</u> of a complete diagnostic assessment for Neuro-Developmental Delay. Reflex inhibition training should only be undertaken after a full assessment and under the supervision of a qualified therapist.

****

SCORING

      A scale of 0 - 4 is used:

      0 = No abnormality detected, i.e. no evidence of
        a primitive reflex, or postural reflex fully developed

      1 = evidence of primitive reflex to 25%
        partial absence of a postural reflex to 25%

      2 = residual presence of a primitive reflex to 50%
        underdeveloped postural reflex to 50%

      3 = virtually retained primitive reflex to 75%
        virtual absence of postural reflex to 75%

      4 = retained primitive reflex, 100% present,
        complete absence of postural reflexes

****

1. Moro Reflex
Standard Test for Vestibular-Activated Moro

Emergence: 9-32 weeks in utero
Birth: fully present
Inhibited: 2-4 months neonate

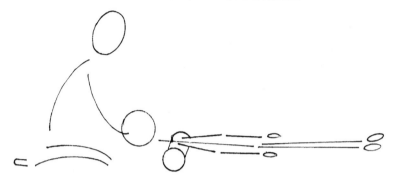

Test position
Supine, with arms flexed and hands resting on the floor. Shoulders should be raised with a small cushion and the child's head supported in the tester's hands and elevated approximately 2 inches above the level of the spine.

Test procedure
After just a few moments the tester should allow the child's head to drop 2-3 inches to just below the level of the spine, but not to reach the floor, having first given the instruction, "When you feel your head drop you must clasp your hands together across your chest as quickly as you can."

Observations
Any movement of the arms outward away from the body. Inability to bring the arms across the chest, or delayed action. Disorientation or distress as a result of the test procedure.

Scoring
0	immediate hand clasp and no adverse reaction
1	slight delay in reaction
2	delayed reaction, incomplete hand/arm movement or breath holding
3	no arm movement, alteration in breathing, and visible dislike of testing procedure
4	movement of the arms outward away from the body, leg extension and/or distress

Also note any reddening of skin or pallor immediately after testing

2. Moro Reflex
Erect Test
(Clarke, Bennett and Rowston)
for
Vestibular-activated Moro

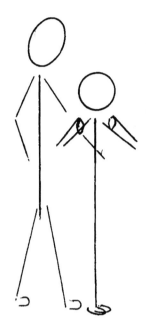

Test Position
Subject stands with feet together,
arms bent and held at 45° from the body
with the hands flexed at the wrists.

Test Procedure
Tester stands behind the subject and instructs the child to put his head
back as if looking at the ceiling and to close his eyes. Note any arm
movement or loss of balance as a result of putting the head into
extension. Once the subject has stabilized in this position, give the
instruction to remain still and fall backwards "like a soldier on parade"
at a given sound. Tester must be prepared to catch the full weight of the
subject.

Observations
Abduction of the arms on falling back and/or intake of breath or cry as
he loses the center of balance. Is there notable reddening of the skin or
pallor, tremor and "withdrawal" immediately after testing?

Scoring

0	subject falls back with no alteration of arm position
1	reddening of the skin or slight but quickly controlled movement of the arms or hands outwards
2	inability to drop back, movement of the arms and hands outwards, dislike of procedure
3	movement of the arms accompanied by "freezing" momentarily in this position, gasp of breath, reddening of the skin or pallor
4	complete abduction of the arms and hands outward accompanied by gasp, freeze and possible cry. Visible dislike or distress

3. Palmar reflex

Emergence: 11 weeks in utero
Birth: present
Inhibited: 2-3 months neonate

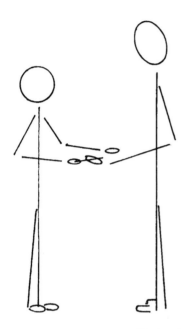

Test position
Standing, feet together with arms bent and palms upturned in a flexed, relaxed position, elbows away from the body.

Test procedure
Gently stroke with a soft brush along the creases of the palm. Repeat twice.

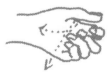

Observations
Any movement of the fingers or thumb inwards toward the stimulus, or extreme sensitivity in the palmar region.

Scoring

0	no response
1	slight movement of the fingers or thumb inward
2	definite movement of the thumb or fingers inward, subject complains touch is ticklish or painful
3	movement of the thumb and/or fingers inward as if to grasp the stimulus, rubbing of the hands immediately after testing
4	thumb and fingers close in on stimulation. This may be accompanied by simultaneous movements of the lips

4. Asymmetrical Tonic Neck Reflex Standard Test
(This test is designed to be used on young babies and may or may not elicit response in an older child who has developed musculature and methods of compensation and control)

Emergence: 18 weeks in utero
Birth: present
Inhibited: 4-6 months of life

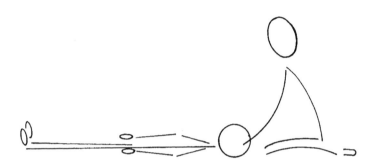

Test position
Supine with arms flexed away from the body and hands resting on finger tips.

Test procedure
Ensure the subject's head is relaxed at the midline. Slowly rotate the head to one side. Hold in that position for 15-20 seconds and observe reactions in arms and legs. Return the head to the midline. Pause for several seconds. Slowly rotate the head to the other side. Pause for 15- 20 seconds. Repeat procedure 3-4 times.

Observations
Note any movement in the body on the side to which the head is turned, particularly in the hand, arm, foot and leg on that side. Any tendency to increased extensor tone on the side to which the head is turned suggests an ATNR might be present. Inability to relax the neck muscles or permit turning of the head beyond a specific point may also suggest a controlled ATNR.

Scoring
0	no response
1	slight tremor in the fingers
2	movement of the hand, arm or leg, or alteration of muscle tone through the torso
3	involuntary extensor movement of any part of the body on the side to which the head is turned, or flexion of the side
4	full extension of the arm and/or leg on the side to which the head is turned with flexion of occipital limbs

5 Asymmetrical Tonic Neck Reflex Schilder Test

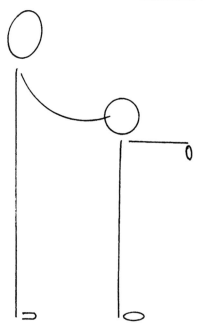

Test position

Standing, feet together, with the arms held straight out at shoulder level and height, but with the hands relaxed at the wrists.

Test procedure

Tester stands behind the subject and gives the instruction: "When I turn your head, I want you to keep your arms straight out in front of you, as they are now. This means your arms remain in the same position, and only your head moves." Tester then slowly rotates the subject's head until the chin is parallel with the shoulder. Pause for 10 seconds. Return the head to the midline. Pause for 10 seconds. Rotate the head to the other side and pause for 10 seconds. Repeat the procedure up to 4 times.

Observations

Any movement of the hand and arm on the side to which the head is turned, i.e. do the arms automatically follow the movement of the head?

Scoring

0	no response
1	slight movement of the arms in the direction the face is pointed
2	movement of the arms in the direction of the head to 45°
3	arm movement to 60° or flexion of the opposite side
4	90° rotation of the arms and/or loss of balance as a result of head rotation

6 Rooting Reflex

Emergence: 24-28 weeks in utero
Birth: present
Inhibited: 3-4 months neonate

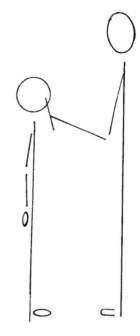

Test position
Standing

Test procedure
Using a small brush, gently stroke from the outer
base of the nose downwards beyond the corner
of the mouth. Repeat two or three times on each side.

Observations
Note any movement or twitching of the mouth in response to the
stimulus, or, withdrawal. Also note any accompanying involuntary
movement of the hands (suggestive of Babkin response).

Scoring
0	no reaction
1	slight twitching of the mouth
2	definite movement of the mouth and/or dislike of the sensation
3	movement and opening of the mouth and/or rubbing of the area stimulated
4	movement of the mouth as if to "smile", opening of the mouth and turning of the head in the direction of the stimulus

7 Suck Reflex

*Repeat procedure as for rooting reflex, but gently stimulate central
area above the upper lip with brush or finger.*

Observations
Involuntary pursing of the lips

Scoring
0	no reaction
1	disproportionate sensation in area stimulated
2	slight movement of the lips
3	pursing of the lips
4	pursing of the lips and tongue movement

8 Spinal Galant Reflex

Emergence: about 20 weeks in utero
Inhibited: 3-9 months of life

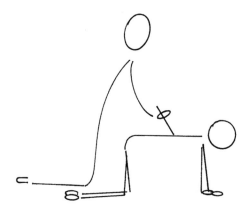

Test position
Four point kneeling or "table" position

Test procedure
Using a light brush, stroke down the back from below the shoulder to
the base of the lumbar region at a distance of 1/2 inch from the spine,
first on one side, then on the other. Repeat the procedure up to 3 times
(repetition beyond this can fail to elicit the reaction even though the
reflex is present).

Observations
Movement of the hip outwards in response to stimulation

Scoring
0   no response
1   undulation or movement of the hip outwards to 15°
2   undulation or movement of the hip outwards to 30°
3   undulation or movement of the hip outwards to 45°
4   movement outwards, beyond 45° and may affect the child's
         balance.

Hypersensitivity—ticklishness—may also be present

9 Tonic Labyrinthine Reflex (Erect Test)

It should be noted that this test only represents one test in a battery of tests for the tonic labyrinthine reflex. (TLR)

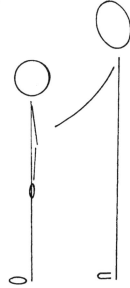

Emerges: Birth
Inhibited: 2-3 months in the prone position,
2-4 months in the supine position, but may still be
present in a weakened form up to the age of 3 years

Test position
Standing with feet together, and arms straight
at the sides of the body.

Test procedure
Slowly tilt the subject's head back into extended position and ask the
subject to close the eyes. (Stand behind to support in case there is any
loss of balance). After 10 seconds ask the subject to slowly move the
head forward as if looking at the toes, and maintain that position for a
further 10 seconds. Repeat the sequence 6 times.

Observations
Note any loss of balance or alteration of balance as a result of head
position, or as a result of head movement from above to below the
level of the spine. Also note any compensatory change in muscle tone
at the back of the knees as a result of head movement, or, gripping with
the toes. Ask the subject for any reactions immediately after testing,
and note any comments about dizziness or nausea, both of which
suggest faulty vestibular functioning and/or the residual presence of the
tonic labyrinthine reflex.

Scoring
0   no response
1   slight alteration of balance as a result of head position or
     movement
2   disturbance of balance during test and/or alteration of muscle
     tone at the back of the knees
3   near loss of balance, alteration of muscle tone and/or
     disorientation as a result of the testing procedure
4   loss of balance and/or massive alteration of muscle tone in
     attempt to maintain balance. This may be accompanied by
     dizziness or nausea, and in adults, feelings of panic

10 Symmetrical Tonic Neck Reflex

Emerges: 6-8 months of life
Inhibited: 9-11 months

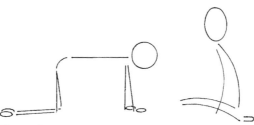

Figure 1

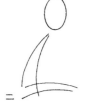

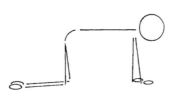

Figure 2

Test position
Four point kneeling "table" position

Test procedure
Subject is instructed to maintain the test position but to slowly move the head to look down "as if looking between your thighs." Hold position for up to 5 seconds and then slowly move the head upwards "as if looking at the ceiling." Repeat up to 6 times.

Observations
Any bending of the arms as a result of head flexion and/or raising of the feet (Fig. 1)

Straightening of the arms and flexion of the knees as a result of head extension (Fig. 2)

Scoring
0   no response
1   tremor in one or both arms or slight hip movement.
2   movement of the elbow on either side and/or definite movement in the hips, or arching of the back
3   bending of the arms on head flexion or movement of the bottom back on head extension
4   bending of the arms to the floor, or movement of the bottom back onto the ankles, so that the subject is sitting in the "cat" position

11 Landau Reflex

Emerges: 2-4 months of life
Inhibited: approximately 3 years of age

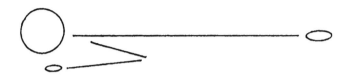

Figure 1

Test position
Prone with arms at right angles to the shoulders (Fig. 1)

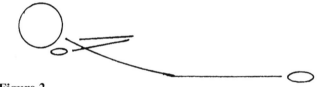

Figure 2

Test procedure
Subject is instructed to lift upper trunk, arms and hands off the floor, keeping feet on the floor, and to maintain elevated position for up to 5 seconds. (Fig.2) This may be repeated twice.

Observations
Involuntary lifting of the feet or lower legs as a result of raising the torso.

Scoring
0   no response
1   slight lifting of one or both feet, immediately corrected
2   definite lifting of one or both feet
3   elevation of both feet away from the floor
4   elevation of both feet several inches above the floor and extensor tone throughout the body

12 Amphibian Reflex

Emergence: 4 - 6 months neonatal
Not inhibited

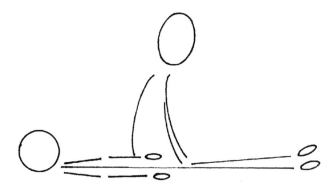

Test position
First supine, then prone.

Test procedure
1. Ensure subject is completely relaxed
2. Tester places hands under hip and elevates it to angle of 45°

Observations
As hip is elevated, knee on same side should bend in both supine and prone testing.

Scoring
0	Knee bends on side of elevated hip
1	No visible flexion of knee, but leg remains relaxed
2	Leg remains stiff
3	Leg is so stiff it begins to lift
4	Whole body rolls rigidly

13 Segmental Rolling Reflex

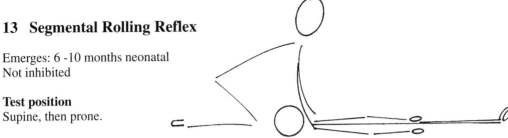

Emerges: 6 -10 months neonatal
Not inhibited

Test position
Supine, then prone.

Test procedure 1
Lift shoulders gently to approximately 45°, at the same time pressing down on the opposite shoulder, and rotate towards opposite side of body.

Observations
As shoulder is lifted, knee on the same side should begin to bend.

Test procedure 2
(Not to be used on cerebral palsy subject.)
Support subject's left heel in left hand.
Apply gentle pressure to bent
left knee with right hand.
Rotate knee slowly across
subject's body until resistance
is met, or the floor is touched.

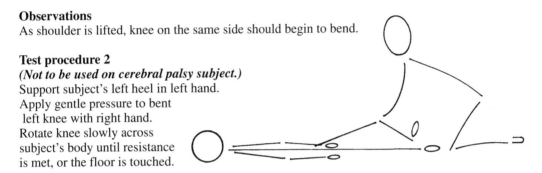

REPEAT PROCEDURE FOR OTHER SIDE.

Observations
Shoulder on same side as rotated knee should begin to lift as knee crosses midline. As knee touches floor, shoulder and arm should follow to complete the rolling over.

Scoring for right and left side separately.

Procedure 1 (Lifting shoulder)
0   Definite bending of knee as shoulder on same side is lifted
1   Tendency for knee to bend, although it does not do so, as shoulder is lifted
2   Leg remains stationary as shoulder on same side is lifted
3   Entire body and leg lift as shoulder on same side is lifted
4   No response at all

Procedure 2 (Pressure on bent knee)
0   Delayed lifting of shoulder, followed by arm and shoulder rolling over to follow knees
1   Incomplete rotation of shoulder
2   Shoulder lifts but does not rotate over completely
3   Slight tendency, as the knee crosses the midline, for the shoulder to lift, or the entire body to rotate
4   No response at all

14 OCULO-HEADRIGHTING REFLEX

Emergence: 2-3 months neonatal
Not inhibited

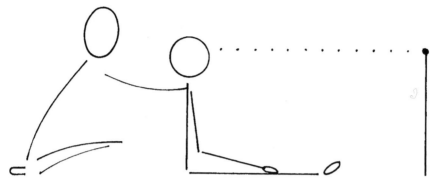

Test Position
Subject seated on floor, legs straight in front, arms resting on thighs.

Test Procedure
1. Subject fixes eyes on an object at eye level.
2. Tester sits behind subject and slowly tilts the subject to the left in 3 stages, pausing for 2 or 3 seconds at each stage. Pauses are made at 15°, 30° and 45°. *Note the position of the subject's head at each degree of tilt.*
3. Return the subject to the upright sitting position, again in the 3 stages.
4. Repeat procedure to the right, return to the midline and then repeat the procedure backwards and forwards, ensuring that the subject keeps the eyes fixed on the object at eye level.

Observations
Head should automatically correct itself to the midline (vertical to the ground) as the body position is altered in all four directions. Any flopping of the head or over-compensation in the opposite direction upon return to the midline position suggests an absent or under-developed oculo-headrighting reflex. Also note any extension of the leg on the side to which the subject is tilted — this may be an indication of a retained asymmetric tonic neck reflex (ATNR) in the leg.

Scoring

0	Head corrects to vertical midline position throughout the test
1	Head slips slightly from the vertical
2	Head follows direction of the tilt in line with the body
3	Head leans below the line of the body
4	Head drops in direction of the tilt

Lack of headrighting forwards/backwards could indicate underlying tonic labyrinthine reflex (TLR).

15 LABYRINTHINE HEADRIGHTING REFLEX

Emergence: 2-3 months neonatal
Not inhibited

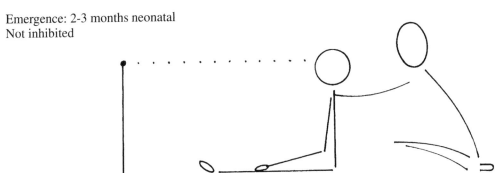

Test Position

Same as for oculo-headrighting reflex, but the subject is asked to fixate his eyes on an object at eye level, and then CLOSE his eyes and to imagine looking at the object during the entire testing procedure.

Test Procedure

1. Subject is instructed to fixate the eyes at eye level object, and then close the eyes and visualize the object throughout the entire testing procedure.
2. Follow the same testing procedure as for oculo-headrighting reflex.

Observations

Note position of the head in all four quadrants, but also note where the subject's closed eyes seem to be directed. (Many children can compensate when their eyes are open, but rapidly lose any sense of where they are in space as soon as the eyes are closed.)

Scoring

0. Head corrects to the vertical midline position throughout the testing
1. Head slips slightly from the vertical
2. Head follows direction of the tilt in line with body
3. Head slips below the line of the body
4. Head drops in the direction of the tilt — no righting apparent

Also note any compensatory turning of the head — this is NOT the same as automatic righting.

Chapter 6

HOW CAN WE HELP?

It is not the aim of this book to turn the readers into therapists, but to give them an understanding of what neurological factors may interfere with a child's progress and what developmental intervention might help. Every child's profile is different and this is where the skill and the training of a therapist becomes necessary when professional help is indicated.

Reflex assessment can be used to identify what type of intervention will be appropriate. Treatment will depend not only upon the severity of the problem but also on the resources—physical conditions, special education experts and remedial programs —available at the school.

You will remember from the chapter on testing that the reflexes are scored using a 5 point scale from 0 to 4. A score of 0 means that no abnormality is present on that particular test. On the other hand, a score of 4 denotes a major problem with that reflex. Most children can compensate if there are traces of abnormality on one or two of the reflexes. If, however, a cluster of abnormal reflexes is in existence, this will affect motor development and motor related skills. A child's score on the reflex test can provide an indication of the type (level) of remediation required.

LEVEL I

If, for example, a child scores higher than 10 on the tests for primitive reflexes, he needs a specific reflex stimulation/inhibition program tailored to his profile. An individual program should only be given following an assessment by a practitioner qualified in the management of a reflex program and progress should be monitored at regular intervals.

LEVEL II

A score of between 8 and 10 on the tests for primitive reflexes together with a score of more than 12 on the postural reflex tests would also indicate benefit from an individualized program.

LEVEL III

Children with scores lower than 8 on either group of reflex tests can benefit greatly from more generalized developmental exercises that can be incorporated into the school day.

All children can benefit from increased opportunity for physical development at home and at school.

How Parents Can Help

Most of us watch in awe as our children grow from helpless babies to walking, talking and determined individuals. As parents we are usually unaware of all the reflexes that play a part in moving from one stage to the next. Growth and development are gradual processes in which reflexes do not simply appear one minute and then disappear the next, but gently change from one to another, often co-existing for a short period of time until the next developmental skill is established.

The word DISCIPLINE means "to teach," hence the word DISCIPLE meaning "pupil." Modern interpretation tends to be dominated by connotations of chastisement, whereas orginally the Latin noun "disciplina" meant instruction or knowledge and later came to be understood as the maintenance of order (necessary to learn) or the provision of an orderly framework within which learning can take place.

Besides love and discipline, freedom to move and freedom to play are two of the most important gifts parents can give to their child. If we want to make sure the baby learns to hold his head up, we put him on his tummy, sit in front of him and talk to him. If he does not want to turn over, we hold something bright to his side, so that he is motivated to turn. To help connect his vestibular system to body awareness, we play "This is the way the ladies ride," or "Down in the deep blue sea." In short, we do all the things that mothers have done instinctively with their children for centuries.

"Children learn most when there is joy in learning." (Kiphard 2000) Young children experience movement with joy and will often peal with laughter when swung through the air, or when they have learned how to roll over they delight in their own developing mobility.

A child's learning begins with his own body. Babies are fascinated by their own body parts and will spend any amount of time intrigued by the movement of their fingers and toes before they realize that these moving objects actually belong to them! A child's earliest exploration of the environment is with his mouth. Through the mouth he learns not only about taste and smell, but also about size, shape and texture. The mouth is furnished with millions of neural connections to the brain that, each time they are being used, help to "map" sensory and spatial information in the brain. The child who is free to explore with his mouth is also free to experiment with sounds and with the cooing, babbling and imitation, which are the genesis of speech.

Movement and vestibular stimulation are experienced as joy. Through movement, a baby can explore the environment and express his emotions (emotion — from the French word *Émouvoir*, meaning *to excite or to move the feelings of*, and *"joy"* which is derived from the French word *"jouer"* meaning *to play*). Posture, muscle tone and facial expression will all alter as the emotional state changes, and sometimes toddlers will utilize earlier reflexes to express their anger or protest.

Have you ever tried to put a toddler into a baby seat when he did not want to go? The body goes rigid as the child accesses the Tonic Labyrinthine Reflex in extension. This makes it impossible to bend his body in the middle and thus helps him to get his own way. As his anger and frustration increase, he will often jerk his head backwards and forwards, strengthening the effect of the reflex and simultaneously working his way into a full-blown tantrum

Modern baby equipment has been a godsend for parents, but molded baby seats, buggies and car seats should never replace the floor as baby's first playground. It is time spent in free play on the floor that helps a child to learn control over his body and therefore gain confidence. On the floor there is freedom to move and to gain experience from different types of exploratory adventures that the child can't have from the confines of a chair.

While lying on the tummy, a baby first learns to hold his head up. A few months later, he will learn how to roll from tummy to back and eventually how to achieve the sitting and crawling positions. In order to sit, a baby must pass through many stages of motor development: He achieves control over posture and gets mastery of balance, each stage heralding increased maturity of the central nervous system. If an adult places the baby in a sitting position, that child cannot pass through these stages spontaneously and may become afraid of falling because he does not know how to retrieve his balance by himself.

With each new achievement, such as having learned to sit up, learned how to get on to hands and knees and having learned to stand up, comes a new problem — having to cope with a new relationship with gravity. Each stage will need practice if automatic balance and coordination are to be acquired. In the first few years of life, practice of motor skills and play are much the same thing.

According to Panksepp (1988) rough and tumble play is the direct result of spontaneous neural urges within the brain and he suggests that it is during play that various neuronal growth factors are recruited. Studies have shown that animals are especially prone to behave in flexible and creative ways and it is thought that games that allow for "rough housing" help in the development of social skills and allow for behavior change. In short, this type of play affords an opportunity to "prime" the limbic system, which is the part of the brain largely responsible for our emotions. This is especially important because it has many connections to the forebrain, which in turn is heavily involved in impulse control and behavior.

Most parents want to protect their children from the dangers of the outside world, but sometimes this can actually prevent them from developing the very skills they need to survive. We learn balance by falling over and then developing strategies to prevent ourselves from falling again. We learn how to tolerate heights by climbing and becoming proficient at it. Most finely honed skills develop out of initial failure and then the desire to overcome the problem. In this sense, early failure is one of life's most important teachers, for it teaches us that we can find new ways to success. Parents who allow their children to test out their environment —within safe boundaries, of course— help their children to grow by allowing them the opportunity to learn by experience. Experience is food for brain development.

A study which examined the incidence of Alzheimer's in an elderly population found a connection between early verbal ability and vocabulary, and the continuation of mental agility towards the end of life. The study was carried out amongst a group of nuns who had had to write a biography of their life prior to entering the convent. These biographies were examined when the nuns were in their 70s, 80s and in some cases 90s. The ones who had demonstrated an extensive vocabulary at the time of entry into the community still had the most alert mental functioning in old age. In addition to educational background, the factor they had in common was that all had been extensively read to when they were children. One of the researcher's conclusions was a message to parents — "Read to your child, read to your child, and when you have finished, read to your child again." (Snowden 2001)

Awareness is half the battle. If for one reason or another reflexes do not mature, we start looking for help.

LEVEL I

Needs professional help

If testing in a child who is over 7 years of age shows that a cluster of primitive reflexes are retained, i.e. a score of more than 9 over 6 tests, then a more detailed reflex and development assessment should be carried out and a specific reflex stimulation/inhibition program devised by a qualified therapist. A score of 3 or 4 on the "big four" reflexes, (ATNR, STNR, TLR, Moro) will have a profound impact on the functioning of the child, whereas a scattered score of 1s and 2s over several reflexes will have a more subtle effect.

A reflex stimulation/inhibition program is tailored to the reflex profile of the individual child. Progress is monitored at regular intervals and the prescribed exercises adjusted accordingly. Reflex stimulation/ inhibition techniques are based upon the theory of replication: i.e. *it is possible to replicate specific stages of early development through the repetition of movement patterns based upon early development.* Reflex stimulation and inhibition movements are based on very early, primitive movements that an older child would not normally make. In this way the brain is given a "second chance" to experience input from the developmental stages that were omitted or incomplete in the first year of life. These stages should have been fundamental in priming the system for later learning, and in recreating them we will establish neural connections and thus reset the neural clock.

When this occurs some children regress both developmentally and emotionally for a short period of time while they are doing such a program. It is therefore important that even though the program is carried out at home, it should only be done with careful guidance and qualified supervision.

A specific reflex stimulation/inhibition program compares to general exercises as a prescription from the pharmacy compares to over-the-counter medication. In fact, "playing" with reflexes without training can do more harm than good, which is why we do not present absolutes in this book.

LEVEL II

Remediation may be done at school or in the home with professional support

It has been determined that if the child has underdeveloped postural reflexes (but only minimal evidence of primitive reflex activity), the child will respond well to a more general program of physical exercises designed to stimulate the postural reflexes and to improve balance and coordination.

> There are many excellent motor training programs available that can be used within the school system: Kephart, Cratty, Dennison (Brain Gym), Lefroy and many more.

> When sensory problems are suspected, there is a program called **Sensory Integration.** *It is based on a system of therapy devised by A. Jean Ayres using sensory input techniques combined with movement to enhance the clarity of incoming information via each of the senses. It strives for efficient transmission of information via the central nervous system (CNS), and the development of more mature patterns of response.*

LEVEL III

Can benefit from a generalized developmental program

For those children who show there is some evidence of primitive reflex activity (a score of 2 or less than 3 on the primitive reflex tests), or in cases where an individualized program is simply not possible, INPP has designed a program of developmental exercises which can be used in school with groups or by a whole class of children over the course of one academic year. This more general program has been piloted in

Germany, Sweden, Ireland and in a number of schools in the United Kingdom. Early results have shown consistent cross cultural improvements, usually beginning with changes in control of balance and coordination (activities such as learning to ride a bicycle, learning to swim and ability to kick, throw and catch a ball), ability to sit still, organization and presentation of work, self confidence, significant improvement in reading and marked improvement in handwriting.

Awareness in the School

When teachers first meet their pupils, they will have had no control over the child's early development. A reflex assessment would be a quick insight into how such a development had occurred and what special needs might have to be met. A specific program of exercises to make sure each child will have the necessary benchmarks needed for success in school would be ideal. Unfortunately such a program is not appropriate for every school. Nevertheless, concepts of development can be incorporated into all levels of teaching. Awareness provides the clues to understanding a child's behavior and is the first step to bringing about change.

TEACHING WITH NORMAL CHILD DEVELOPMENT IN MIND

Once the universality and mechanics of normal development are understood, a suitable program of motor and sensory stimulation can be put together — either for the individual child or for the whole class. As a general guide, normal development follows a set sequence: Motor development begins in a cephalo-caudal (from head to toe) and proximo-distal (from the center outwards) pattern. Sensory development begins with the vestibular and tactile systems and is closely followed by auditory, visual and proprioceptive development. None of these systems function independently. Any attempt at physical remediation should take this normal pattern of development into account.

The next chart is a model which provides a framework in which to see how various systems in early development interact to provide a basis for later learning. At the bottom of the figure are some of the early influences which will affect the development of the child. These early ingredients are like the roots of the tree. If the roots are strong and firmly established, the tree has a good foundation from which to grow.

Amongst the roots is the vestibular system, the only one of the sensory systems to be myelinated by the time of birth. After birth, the balance mechanism must learn how to interact with the other developing sensory systems: touch, vision, hearing, etc. In the early weeks of life the sensory systems are entrained and integrated through usage: through movement and interaction with the environment. The primitive reflexes provide a mechanism with which the neonate can respond to sensation through movement. In this context, the primitive reflexes form the base of the trunk of the tree from which the branches (the developing cortex) will later benefit.

As the primitive reflexes are inhibited in the first 6-12 months of life and are replaced by postural reflexes, so the trunk of the tree that carries neurological connections between the brain and the body grows stronger. At the same time that these changes are taking place, the cerebellum passes through its first major stage of maturation.

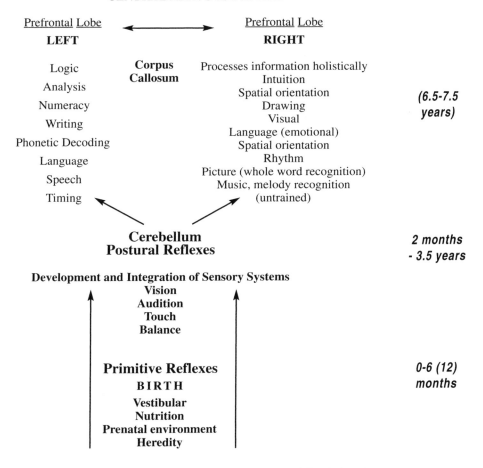

THE TREE OF DEVELOPMENT
STAGES OF MATURATION IN THE
CENTRAL NERVOUS SYSTEM

Prefrontal Lobe ⟷ Prefrontal Lobe
LEFT **RIGHT**

Logic	**Corpus Callosum**	Processes information holistically
Analysis		Intuition
Numeracy		Spatial orientation
Writing		Drawing
Phonetic Decoding		Visual
Language		Language (emotional)
Speech		Spatial orientation
Timing		Rhythm

(6.5-7.5 years)

Picture (whole word recognition)
Music, melody recognition
(untrained)

Cerebellum
Postural Reflexes

2 months - 3.5 years

Development and Integration of Sensory Systems
Vision
Audition
Touch
Balance

Primitive Reflexes
BIRTH
Vestibular
Nutrition
Prenatal environment
Heredity

0-6 (12) months

Both hemispheres of the cerebral cortex also mature rapidly during the first months and years of life and continue to gain increased control over lower centers. **Until approximately 7 years of age, the right hemisphere is slightly ahead of the left** *(see chapter 3)*, **and for certain skills the right hemisphere acts like a training ground for the left. The right hemisphere is particularly good at learning batteries of information through music, rhythm and movement or, put another way, at learning** *with* **the body.**

A generation ago —in fact throughout history— it was fairly standard practice to start teaching children younger than seven years old the alphabet and multiplication tables, but only to music or rhymes. The younger child did not necessarily understand the meaning of what it had learned until later, but the information once learned was filed away, available to be accessed at a later stage when required. Changing trends in educational theory threw out some of these "out-dated" modes of teaching, asserting that a child needs to understand the meaning of numbers before multiplication tables are relevant. The result has been that many children do not start learning their tables until 8 years of age or above. **It is just at this developmental stage that the child should be transferring more direct learning to the left hemisphere and the left hemisphere does not find it easy to learn batteries of information in this way. Many children above 8 years of age struggle to learn their tables even though they may have some understanding of the meaning of multiplication.** *(It is important to remember that at school entrance girls are about six months ahead in this development and not to expect the same performance from boys as from girls.)*

Learning by rote before 7 years of age coincides with a time of developmental readiness when the right hemisphere is particularly receptive to stimulation through movement, rhyme and song. The cerebellum is also maturing rapidly during these years and the research of Leiner, Leiner, Dow and others (1986) has shown the cerebellum also to be active during rote learning. It would appear that the learning of new skills is most easily absorbed if it coincides with the time of appropriate brain development sometimes referred to as "the window of opportunity" or the time of neurological readiness.

Children can learn the alphabet to a tune at a younger age and then store that information to be applied at a later stage when the rules of phonetic decoding and spelling are required. Alan Schore (1994) suggests that learning and development are a continuous process of interaction between the two hemispheres with one hemisphere being dominant at one stage of learning and the other hemisphere taking over later on. In this way, both hemispheres are involved in the learning process but eventually one should take precedence over the other for specific tasks. Art, music and physical education are the other half of language. Children who suffer from neuro-developmental delay are often still "stuck" at an earlier phase of development and benefit from being allowed to "retrace" some of the earlier stages of learning key skills.

SENSORY DIFFICULTIES
Einstein said that all life forms share the characteristic of movement. Of the senses crucial to learning, five share the perception of motion as a common denominator. Where there is motion, there is frequency. Balance, touch, hearing, vision and proprioception are all the result of response to movement at varying frequencies or through a different medium. The vestibular system responds to slow movement (the

maximum stimulation for the vestibular system is 1° of an arc per second (Guyton 1991). The sense of touch is felt as a result of movement across the hair cells located in the dermis of the skin, or by pressure applied to the skin. Low frequency sound is sometimes "felt" through the tactile system as vibrations and only as the frequency of vibrations per second (hz) increases does the sense of hearing take over in the perception of sound. Vision is the brain's response to the movement of light photons at a higher frequency still. The ability to "make sense" of movement through the sensory systems is the foundation of learning. The first system in development to answer the call of movement is the vestibular system.

BALANCE — THE BEGINNING OF PRAXIS

Balance is not something that happens to us, it is something that we do. It is an adaptive complex behavior that results from a series of abilities against **imbalance**. Functional balance makes it possible to perform useful actions while maintaining a certain position. This is the foundation for praxis (action). In this way, exercises that improve balance through stimulation of the vestibular system can improve praxis, orientation and behavior (Schrager 2001).

Praxis:
The brain's ability to select responses, arrange them in an appropriate order and orient them for proper execution.

The most advanced level of movement is the ability to stay totally still and perfect balance is the action of not moving (Rowe 1996). Movement helps matter to maintain balance over a narrow base of support. Remember learning how to ride a bicycle? Initially, balance could only be maintained once the bicycle was in motion, and the faster you went, the better your balance seemed to be. The hardest part was learning to start and stop without falling off when movement slowed down. As your control over the center of balance improved, so less speed was needed to retain control. Children who have difficulty sitting still often have immature control over balance. They are still at a stage when they need to be "on the move" to function. In school we require our children to sit still for long periods of time. Those children who fidget and lose concentration after 15-20 minutes often concentrate better for the remainder of the class if they are allowed to get up and move around for a couple of minutes — even in the middle of the lesson. For children with poor balance, movement is food for the brain. Some children will need help to develop new types of movement experience in order to gain better control and an improved vocabulary of movement. This is where the teacher can help.

Dyspraxia (or apraxia) is the inability to do so even though no paralysis exists.

Opportunities for vestibular training can be included in the school day and do not necessarily have to be confined to physical education classes. With any exercise regime, the best results are achieved if exercises are practiced daily rather than being confined to a 40 minutes class, once a week.

EXAMPLES OF VESTIBULAR STIMULATION
The vestibular system functions on three planes:
1. Horizontal head rotation about a vertical axis (z axis = yaw)
2. Head extension and flexion about a horizontal axis
   (y axis = pitch)
3. Lateral head tilt about a horizontal axis (x axis = roll)

Types of stimulation to each one of these planes would include:

Horizontal stimulation - spinning in an upright position

Rocking — forwards and backwards
swinging forwards and backwards
forward rolls

Lateral — rolling along a horizontal surface

The following types of stimulation are naturally a part of activities and games that involve changes of movement in space:

1. Up and down (vertical) —jumping, hopping, sliding, see-sawing
2. To and fro —running, stopping
3. Centrifugal force —carousel
4. Turning movements of the body such as those used in dance, particularly folk or country dancing
5. Depth —propulsion of the body above the ground eg. scooter board

(Kiphard 2000)

These types of movement experiences can be incorporated into a normal school day.

AUDITORY

The child who has problems in auditory processing will often respond to sound therapy.

It is important to remember that a child may not have a processing problem, but may never have been exposed to the vocabulary itself. If we were to go into a country whose language is foreign to us we would not suddenly have an auditory problem. It would be simply lack of exposure to connecting objects and symbols to specific sounds.

An increasing number of methods are currently available, all of which operate upon a common principle that language skills such as speech, reading, writing, spelling and musical expression can only develop if the child has learned to "listen." Advanced listening involves both the exclusion of irrelevant sounds and the ability to focus upon a specific sound. In this respect, effective listening resembles good vision. The following list is only intended as a guide to help decide which method may be relevant for a particular child:

a) Dyslexia, reading, spelling and articulation difficulties: Auditory Discrimination Training —Dr. Kjeld Johansen, Paul Madaule
b) Autism, aphasia, language and general learning difficulties: Auditory Integrative Training —Dr. Guy Berard

Vestibular stimulation can be calming or alerting. Gentle motion such as rocking or the movement of the car may send us to sleep. More vigorous stimulation such as a roller coaster ride has an excitatory effect. Some children are hyper or hypo in their response to stimulation in one of the vestibular planes.

c) Listening, language and general learning difficulties, the need to fine-tune musical skills and relieve unexplained anxiety:
> The Tomatis Method— individual centers
> Samonas center—Dr. I. Steinbach

Johansen's, Steinbach's and Madaule's systems can be used within school or home environment.

While the above mentioned systems of sound therapy help to improve auditory processing through auditory stimulation, the Tomatis system and Madaule's adaptation of the Tomatis method include exercises which help to train the auditory-vocal feedback loop. Madaule describes listening as "a hidden skill behind learning" and voice as the closing link in the loop between the individual and the environment. It is the completion of this loop that enables a person to become self-sufficient by connecting linguistically to the outside world.

AUDITORY PROCESSING AND LEARNING

The auditory system processes several types of information:
1. Vibration (with the tactile system)
2. Sound
3. Rhythm (with vestibular system)
4. Timing (with vestibular system)
5. Orientation in space. While vision gives us forward spatial awareness, hearing helps us to be aware of what is happening behind and around us.

Efficient auditory processing is dependent upon:
1. Adequate hearing levels/auditory discrimination
2. Direct transmission of information to the appropriate area in the brain (laterality)
3. Speed of transmission. Individuals labeled dyslexic often process the sounds of speech more slowly than the norm (Shaywitz 1996, Tallal, 1996)
4. Ability to shut out irrelevant sounds

What are some of the stages in early development that a child passes through as it develops auditory processing skills?
1. Continuous exposure to the sounds of the mother tongue
2. Language heard without background noise
3. Vocalization and action; vocalization and response
4. Stage of subvocalization— As young children start to learn something they very often carry on a personal monologue. This process of vocalization helps to embed material into memory through the stages of perception, expression, repetition and recognition. The *doing* stage (vocalization) helps to pass information to the language center in the left hemisphere of the cortex. As we mature, we learn to "internalize" this voice, and we may use our "inner voice" to help solve problems.

What else other than sound therapy can be done to improve auditory processing?

1. Regular "sounding out" as a class
2. Using song, rhyme and movement to aid memorization of material (what I know in my body, I know in my head)
3. Use of song to slow down the sounds of speech

Paula Tallal has devised a computer-based training program that artificially slows down the sounds of speech to allow the child time to hear each sound within a word. Setting words to music has a similar effect. Each syllable within a word is given accent, time (spatial dimension) and tonal value, so that a simple sentence such as,

Early one morning, just as the sun was rising,

is sung as

Ear-ly one mo-o-r--ning, just as the sun was ri-i-sing . . .

This elongates the time factor in the enunciation of sounds, which in turn helps the child to register and articulate individual sounds in each word. Children with spelling problems often spell exactly as they hear, so that a word like "remember" may be written as "rembr." The middle syllable within the word has not been registered auditorally.

4. Create an external feedback loop to improve the ear-voice connection. Madaule suggests cupping the right hand in front of the mouth and speaking into it. This creates an external resonance chamber that transmits vibrations back to the right ear through bone conduction and encourages more efficient right eared listening.

MUSIC AS A PRIMARY TEACHER

Music can be used to help develop listening acuity, language skills and timing. Music is language without words. In common with other languages, it imposes order, structure, rhythm, timing and sound frequency discrimination on random sound. It gives meaning to sound. In terms of both evolution and development, music can be understood at the most primitive levels, for music is processed at all levels in the brain.

Music is one of life's earliest natural teachers. Before birth, the fetus reacts to music with changes in motor activity; infants respond to music and can imitate simple rhythms before they develop speech. The early cooing of the baby has melody, intonation and cadence, and even in the absence of musical training is perceived primarily by the right side of the brain, the side of the brain responsible for melody recognition, language comprehension, picture recognition, spatial orientation and rhythm. Even though reading does not become proficient until both sides of the brain work together, these are the very skills that the young child needs when *starting* to learn to read. Nursery rhymes, songs and movement to music can all be used in the first five to seven years of life to develop other skills in preparation for literacy.

Just as language and dialect vary from one region of the world to another, so music carries within it the color and flavor of the region from which it grows. Hence, although there are common elements in the folk tunes of the world, there are also language characteristics that are unique to the area of orgin. In this sense, the native language and the music of an area share a common accent. Musical activities give a child a second chance to learn accurate codification and tonal quality of language. This is true even for children who may have suffered intermittent hearing loss in the early years, a time generally considered to be essential for the "fine tuning in" to the sounds of language that are so important for later verbal and literacy skills.

Rhythm begins with the body; it's a vestibular function. Emile Jacques Dalcroze, a professor of Harmony at the Conservatoire of Geneva in the 1890s, noticed that many of his music students were unable to appreciate the chords that they had to write. It was as if they could not hear inside their heads what they had written with their hands. This is similar to difficulties experienced by children with reading and spelling difficulties who are unable to match the phonetic features of a word to the visual symbol. Dalcroze concluded that his students had not had sufficient *physical* experience of chords at the beginning of their studies at the time when brain and body are developing along similar lines. He concluded that in order to overcome this problem *"the ear must gradually accustom itself to grasp the relations between notes, and the **whole body** —by means of special exercises— must be initiated into the appreciation of rhythmic, dynamic and agogic nuances of music."*

Agogic: state of eager excitement or merriment.

Dalcroze developed a series of physical exercises put to music that were designed to develop the inner hearing and musicality of the child through the **use of the body** as a musical instrument. This provided the basis for the Dalcroze approach that can be taught to music teachers for use within schools today. By harnessing a child's natural movements such as walking, running, hopping, skipping, rocking, bending and stretching, the fundamentals of rhythm, rhythmic patterns and phrasing can be taught (Middlemiss 1987). These are also important elements of language.

In the monastic schools of the middle ages, music formed an integral part of education. *"To medieval thinkers, arithmetic, the science of number, was fundamental. Music was the expression of number in time, giving pitch, duration, rhythm, stress and accent to the words. Language regulated by number was song. Number structuring space was geometry."* (Le Mée 1964) In this sense, music can also supply the architecture for many aspects of learning.

Certain sound frequencies have the ability to alter brain wave states. There are four major brainwave states that take us through our cycles of waking and sleeping, relaxation and arousal, lethargy and creativity:

• Beta waves (13 - 22 Hz) keep us in an alert waking state, focused on our external environment. (It has been found that the beta brain waves do not fire consistently at a fast enough rate in some children with ADD and ADHD, hence their difficulty focusing and maintaining attention).

- Alpha waves (8 - 12 Hz) active in states of relaxed consciousness, such as when daydreaming.
- Theta waves (4 - 7 Hz) are active at times of optimum creativity, during deep meditation and when drifting off to sleep.
- Delta waves (.5 - 3.5 Hz) are found in the deepest phase of the sleep cycle and in unconsciousness.

Different combinations of sound and rhythm can both mimic and induce the frequencies that are active in different brain wave states. Music and sound therapy can help to attune the brain to a more desirable frame of mind, depending on the state we want to induce. Many of us subconsciously use this process in the music we select at different times in the day. "Baroque music such as Vivaldi, Bach and Handel has a strong intellectual component and is related to the head, although the rhythm affects our active principle and the timbre and sonority our emotions. Mozart's music seems to provide food for all three principles whilst some rock and roll music that makes the pelvis gyrate hardly moves above the belt." (Le Mée 1994)

A teacher accidentally utilized this effect when she started to play Mozart as background music during her high school science classes. She observed that the general noise level of a normally disruptive class dropped, concentration and behavior improved. To back up her observations, she also had the children's blood pressure measured, both before and after the class in which the Mozart had been played. The blood pressure of the students was consistently lower after the classes in which background classical music had been present. This is not to suggest that classical music should be played as a backdrop to every class. Some children will find it as distracting as others find it helpful, but classical music can be used to improve concentration and enhance creativity under certain conditions. (London Times Education Supplement 1998)

Music lessons can also be used to teach simple exercises that involve listening and vocalization. Play two notes and then teach the child to "hear" which one is higher using movements up and down an imaginary staircase. Help them to judge the interval between two notes. Do two notes played together clash or harmonize? What is the difference in interval between sounds which blend and sounds which clash? Even if the child cannot sing in tune, encourage the child to sing each note, record it on a tape recorder and then modify his singing after listening to the sound of his own voice. Encourage the singing of simple rhymes and sequences to tunes e.g. days of the week, months of the year, tables, alphabet, tongue twisters, etc.

An entire system of general teaching is now available based upon the concept of the "selfvoice". The system ARROW, which is an acronym for Aural-Reading-Respond-Oral-Written requires the child to read a section of text into a special tape recorder. He has to listen to the sound of his own voice, then to rewind and use his own voice to dictate. He also writes down the relevant information. Vast improvements in reading and spelling age are noticeable after only a few weeks of use.

For many children, simply providing a tune can act as a code to a memory filing system and help in both the laying down and the retrieval of information to and from memory storage. These are only a few preliminary ideas upon which more sophisticated exercises can be based.

VISUAL PROCESSING

The range of problems a child might experience with visual processing was outlined in Chapter 3. Symptoms observable in the classroom may include:

- Loss of place following a line of print
- Need to finger-point to maintain visual fixation
- Frequent mistakes when copying
- Flat, monotonous voice when reading aloud
- Poor reading comprehension
- Inability to draw accurately
- Misalignment of columns in arithmetic
- Difficulty catching a ball

Many visual problems will need professional investigation and may involve a visit to:

- An Optician to check visual acuity
- An Orthoptist who may be able to recommend special glasses or eye exercises
- A Developmental or Behavioral Optometrist

Eyesight should always be checked before any other exercises are attempted, even if a profile of abnormal reflexes is known to be present.

If eyesight is found to be normal, but there is a cluster of abnormal reflexes, a reflex stimulation/inhibition program can make a profound difference to both oculo-motor and visual-perceptual skills. A vision therapist working in The Netherlands found that he achieved the greatest success if he delayed using vision therapy until a child had had at least 6 months on a reflex stimulation/inhibition program. In many cases, vision therapy was not required after the reflexes had matured. In those cases where residual oculo-motor problems remained, the time needed on a vision therapy program was halved. (Ten Hoopen 1995)

Until other methods of therapy have succeeded in improving the child's vision, teachers can help to reduce the effect of some visual problems in a number of ways. For children who have tracking problems:

> To help maintain visual fixation on the correct line, allow them to use a ruler under the line. A rectangular "window" cut into a small

piece of cardboard will allow them to concentrate on a few words at a time. This can also help the child who is visually "stimulus bound" and who cannot cope with a lot of visual information presented at one time.

Creating a better environment
in which the child with NDD can learn

The class teacher is usually too busy with the daily curriculum to focus individual attention on the child with neuro-developmental delay (NDD). Signs of some retained reflexes, however, are not only easy to spot, but with the awareness gained from reading the material in Chapters 2 and 3, they are almost impossible to miss. There are always a variety of skill levels seen in a classroom. The following ways will make it easier to adjust teaching methods to the needs of each child. Table III has suggestions, which may be used by all teachers, but the following strategies outlined by Jane Field (1992) may also help to accommodate the NDD child in the classroom.

1. Moro Reflex

Remembering that a child with a retained Moro is the child who over-reacts to almost all stimuli, the most important accommodation that a teacher can make for such a child is to create a classroom with as non-threatening an environment as possible. This can be done by keeping noise levels to a minimum: both her own and that of the children. General movement during teaching should be reduced as much as possible, so that the eyes are more able to attend selectively to what is of immediate concern to them. Careful planning can seat certain children in positions where much of the general bustle of the classroom is outside their field of vision.

All children hate to be singled out —to be different— unless that difference increases status with their peers. The child with a Moro reflex already feels at variance with others and has difficulty fitting into a group. As a result his self-esteem is usually low, or at best, fragile. A teacher who is aware of such a trait and understands the underlying reason, can do much to build confidence without making the child feel conspicuous.

2. Asymmetrical Tonic Neck Reflex

The child who still has an ATNR needs extra space to write in order to accommodate the effect of the reflex. This is the child who may rotate the page as much as 90 degrees to allow for the fact that every time he turns his head to write, his arm wants to stretch. He often pushes the paper to the far side of the working surface particularly when writing near the bottom of the page. Seating a right- and left-handed child together at a table will cause enormous problems for this child. If, in addition, the child also has retained a Moro reflex, then the distractions of "group teaching" may make concentration impossible for him. Simple changes such as arranging the classroom for at least some individual desks or placing tables in rows facing the teacher, will help to minimize distraction and allow each child maximum personal space.

Difficulty with the physical act of writing will prevent the child from being able to express ideas in written form while it is easy for him to do so orally. Ideas can be reinforced by allowing a period of discussion which can then be condensed into key words or phrases as an outline for an essay or a short piece of creative writing. Similarly, the child can be taught to underline salient points. When he is given a paragraph meant to test his comprehension or that is part of an exam question, this will allow him instant access or referral to the main points for discussion.

Use of a laptop computer can aid spelling, grammar and content, as the finger control required for keyboard skills is different from that required for handwriting. Posture and movement at the keyboard do not trigger the ATNR and so the computer frees the child from the physical constraints of the ATNR. Spellchecks can help to reinforce correct spelling and thereby develop better visual-memory for how words should look. Not all children, however, can master the visual-motor integration skills needed for fast and accurate typing (some children with Dyspraxia find this particularly difficult) and in these cases, a computer will only be of limited assistance.

Where improvement in handwriting is essential, some of a child's homework may be done on a computer, and then the correct version copied by hand into the exercise book. This, in effect, separates out the two processes of cognitively processing information and physically writing it down.

3 . Symmetrical Tonic Neck Reflex

This is the child whose posture will be affected by any movement of his head forwards or backwards. This will be particularly noticeable when the child sits at a desk, as inclining the head forward to focus on work will cause the arms to bend and the head to fall nearer and nearer to the working surface. The effect of this can be minimized by altering the angle of the work surface so that the head can be maintained in a more upright posture. The old-fashioned sloping desks were ideal for this, but a triangular structure which can be placed on top of the table will have the same effect.

The effects of the symmetrical tonic neck reflex (STNR) will usually diminish quickly if a motor training program is given.

4. Spinal Galant

The description of effects of the retained Spinal Galant is that it creates an "ants in the pants" child. There are other reasons why a child can't stay in his seat, yet some teachers have found it possible to stop the constant complaints and reminders to keep children still. The main offenders in the classroom are given flat, plastic pillows filled with water. Such simple devices give them enough wriggle room so that they can stay in their seats, and peace and quiet will be restored.

Sometimes even after reflex abnormalities have been corrected a child continues to have problems with integration of the two sides of the body. Independent use of the left and right hands, use of opposite hand and foot, etc., will be difficult. These movement disabilities reflect the inability of the two sides of the brain to co-operate in facilitation, inhibition and transmission of information back and forth across the corpus callosum. Efficient communication between the two cerebral hemispheres in both directions is necessary for all academic learning, particularly for solving problems that require a sequence of procedures. (Solving one simple multiplication problem involves at least nine interactions between the two sides of the brain.)

Sheila Dobie and colleagues at The Institute for Neuro-Physiological Psychology in Scotland have developed a series of exercises that help to train different parts of the body to operate with each other in any number of combinations and sequences. As a child's movement vocabulary increases, basic movement patterns become automatic. Not only does the child's motor competency improve, but corresponding cognitive abilities also show greater flexibility and improved performance.

This is rather like preparing the ground for planting. For a time after seeds have been spread, no visible growth occurs. This is the period of germination, of forming roots below the ground upon which later growth will depend.

Chart III has many further suggestions for those who are in a position to do more than is usually possible in the classroom.

When a child is experiencing difficulties it is often tempting to try to provide the maximum stimulation and support. A study by Kavale and Matson (1983) suggests that if too many types of intervention are done at the same time, the results are less than chance. In other words, there is no significant improvement.

The brain can only take in a certain amount of new information at one time and often needs time to absorb and integrate new information. It is therefore advisable to start with only one method of intervention at a time and allow time to assess progress before building anything further into the program. If the child's behavior starts to deteriorate shortly after something new has been added, this may be a sign that he is "overloaded" and the amount of stimulation needs to be decreased. More is not necessarily better.

DEVELOPMENT AND TRANSFORMATION OF THE REFLEX SYSTEM

REFLEX	EMERGES	INHIBITION	TRANSFORMATION
1. Uterine withdrawal reflexes	5-7 weeks in utero	9-32 weeks in utero	Moro reflex
2. Moro reflex	9-12 weeks in utero	2-4 months neonate	Adult 'startle' response (Strauss reflex)
3. Palmar reflex	11 weeks in utero	2-3 months neonate	Voluntary release progressing to a 'pincer' grip
4. Plantar reflex	11 weeks in utero	7-9 months neonate	Adult Plantar
5. Asymmetrical Tonic Neck reflex	c. 18 weeks in utero	3-9 months neonate	Transformed tonic neck reflex
6. Spinal Galant reflex	20 weeks in utero	3-9 months neonate	Amphibian reflex
7. Rooting reflex and 8. Suck reflex	24-28 weeks in utero	3-4 months neonate	Adult suck reflex and subsequent development of mature sucking and swallowing movements essential for speech and clear articulation
9. Tonic labyrinthine reflex forwards	12 weeks in utero	3-4 months neonate	Headrighting reflex Landau reflex
10. TLR-backwards	Emerges at birth	2-4 months neonate	Headrighting reflexes
11. Babinski reflex	1 week neonate	12-24 months	Adult Plantar
12. Stepping reflex	1 week neonate	6 months	Inhibited by 6 months at the latest
13. Abdominal reflex	4 weeks neonate	remains	Is indicative of increasing maturity in the upper pyramidal tract and thus is associated with balance and muscle tone
14. Landau reflex	4-6 weeks neonate	3 years	Control of balance between flexor and extensor muscles
15. Headrighting reflexes	2-4 months	remains	The basis of balance, oculomotor functioning orientation and spatial awareness

Table I
Table II

HISTORICAL INDICATORS OF NEURO-DEVELOPMENTAL DELAYS

PREGNANCY _____

- Hyperemesis (severe sickness)
- Severe viral infection during the first
  12 weeks or between 26 and 30 weeks
- Excessive alcohol consumption and/or
  drug abuse
- Radiation
- Accident or infection

- Threatened miscarriage
- Hypertension
- Placental insufficiency (small for dates)
- Smoking
- Toxoplasmosis
- Severe stress
- Uncontrolled diabetes

BIRTH _____

- Prolonged labor or precipitive labor
- Placenta previa
- High forceps or ventouse extraction
- Breech
- Cesarian

- Cord around the neck
- Fetal distress
- Premature (more than 2 weeks early) or
  post mature (more than 2 weeks late)

NEWBORN DISORDERS _____

- Low birth weight (under 5 lbs.)
- Incubation
- Distorted skull
- Prolonged jaundice

- Requiring rescusitation
- Blue baby
- Heavy bruising
- Problems with feeding the first 6 months

INFANCY _____

- Illnesses involving a high fever, delirium or
  convulsions in the first 18 months
- Adverse reaction to any of the innoculations
- Late at learning to walk (later than 18 months)
- Late at learning to talk (later than 18 months)

CHILDHOOD & SCHOOL HISTORY _____

- Travel sickness—headache or nausea, especially
  while reading in car, boat or plane.
- Difficulty learning to ride a two wheel bicycle
- Difficulty learning to read
- Difficulty learning to write, or in making the
  transition from printing to cursive script
- Difficulty in learning to tell the time (clock face
  v. digital clock)
- Poor hand-eye coordination

Rarely will a single factor by itself indicate Neuro-Developmental Delay. As with primitive reflexes,
it is only where a cluster of factors exist that NDD may be present. Indicators of NDD are not limited
to the above list.

TABLE III

REMEDIATION FOR RETAINED REFLEXES

Reflex	School Problem	Remediation Approach

Moro Reflex
Test:
1. Head drop in supine
2. Drop back test
	Over-reactive
	Hypersensitive
	Stimulus bound
	Difficulty with ball games
		Sensory: Vestibular training,
		  tactile stimulation,
		  sound therapy

Palmar Reflex Test: 1. Stimulation of the palm of the hand	Poor manual dexterity Immature pencil grip Speech and hand move- ments may be connected	Exercises: A) Clasping and unclasping of the hand around an object; B) Independent thumb movement pro- gressing to thumb opposition and finger movements; C) Finger exercises with hands separately and then making different movements with hands together.
Asymmetrical Tonic Neck Reflex Test: 1. Supine, head rotation 2. Schilder test	Handwriting; expression of ideas in written form; eye tracking problems; Dif- ficulty crossing the midline; ambilaterality or cross laterality	1) Slow exercises which begin with homolateral movements of the body in response to head rotation in same direction while lying supine; Progress to extension of one side of body in opposite direction to head rotation; Independent cross pattern move- ment of arms and legs with head at midline. These should be performed in slow motion while lying on the back. 2) Develop eye tracking movements by asking the child to slowly move the thumb of the dominant hand from side-to-side at a distance of 8-10" from the face, keeping the head still while focusing on the thumb. First, ask the child to do this with eyes closed, imag- ining he is focusing on his thumb, six times, then repeat with the eyes open. 3) Slowly move thumb back and forth from near- point to arm's length while focusing on thumb. Extend the distance of focus to a spot on the wall and then back to the thumb again at arm's length and near-point.
Rooting and Suck Test: Stimulation of the two sides of the mouth.	Poor articulation, prolonged thumb sucking, messy eating, dribbling; oversensitive to touch on the face; possible need for orthodontic treatment later; Swallowing movements too near the front of the mouth may develop a high palate and narrow jaw.	Reflex Inhibition Program
Spinal Galant Test: Stimulation of the lumbar region.	Inability to sit still or remain silent; poor concentration; continued bed wetting above the age of 5 years.	Reflex Inhibition Program if present with other primitive reflexes. If it is the only retained primitive reflex, exer- cises done lying on the back will inhibit the pelvic tilting.
Tonic Labyrinthine Test: Movement of the head through the vertical plane, forward and backward beyond the midline.	Poor balance; rigid or floppy muscle (seen in P.E. when running); oculo-motor dysfunctions: a) tracking, b) convergence, c) reestablish- ment of binocular vision. Visual-perceptual difficul- ties. Possible auditory prob- lems. Organizational problems, poor sense of time and rhythm.	1) Vestibular stimulation, ie. rotation, rolling and rocking, initially done with the eyes closed; 2) Stretching and flexion exercises performed on the floor in supine and prone with eyes closed TLR present above a test score of 2 in conjunction with any other reflex inhibition exercises.

TABLE III *(continued)*

REMEDIATION FOR RETAINED REFLEXES

Reflex	School Problem	Remediation Approach
Symmetrical Tonic Test: Head extension and flexion in table position.	Posture: lies on desk when writing. Poor eye-hand co-ordination; problems with refocusing from far to near distance. Clumsy.	Creeping on hands and knees; provide a sloping or tilted desk surface.
Posturals — Absent or under-developed:		
Headrighting Test:	Oculo-motor dysfunctions, visual-perceptual difficulties. Poor spatial awareness. Motion sickness.	Vestibular training, eg. slow rotation (eyes closed), rolling and tilting, progressing to eyes open as balance and headrighting improves. Scooter board, wobble board, first lying, then sitting, then standing; and using trampoline.
Landau Reflex Test:	Imbalance between extensor and flexor muscles.	Prone — lifting torso off the ground while keeping feet on the ground.
Amphibian and Segmental Rolling Test:	Lack of segmental or differentiated movement through the body.	Rolling from prone to supine and vice-versa, initiating movement from one portion of the body, i.e. bend one leg and slowly bring across the body to stimulate rolling of upper portion of body.
Equilibrium Reactions		These will only develop fully if the Moro and Tonic Labyrinthine reflexes are inhibited; absence of equilibrium reactions may be symptomatic of other retained primitive reflexes.

Chapter 7

The Evolution of an Idea - Reflecting on Reflexes

The word reflex is a derivative of the word "reflection," which etymologically means to "bend it back." The earliest use of the term in this context can be traced back to Thomas Willis (1621-1675) who was one of the first medical physiologists in the seventeenth century to place his faith in clinical and laboratory observation as opposed to the theory of the "humors" and the philosophies of the Greco-Roman tradition. Willis (1670) used the terms "motus reflexus" and "reflex-ion" to describe how impulses or "spirits" in the nerves to the central nervous system could be "reflected" back to the muscles. The automatic action generated by the process was similar to the action of light bouncing off a mirror. It was also Willis who gave us such modern medical terms as "neurology," "lobe" and "hemisphere" (Finger, S. 2000).

The term reflex reappeared in the eighteenth century when Georg Prochaska of Vienna (1784) described, "the reflexion of sensorial into motor impressions . . . which takes place in the common sensory center and which may take place with consciousness or without." Roger Whytt (1751) carried out experiments on animals and attempted to list the functional relationship between reflexes and protective behaviors. He was intrigued by the continued motor activity of animals following decapitation, a well known, but not understood phenomenon. This is woven into the seventeenth century English children's rhyme, "King Charles walked and talked for five minutes after his head was cut off!"

In the 1820s Charles Bell and Francoise Magendie recognized that "between the brain and the muscle there is a circle of nerves; one conveys the influence of the brain to the muscle, another gives the sense of condition of the muscle to the brain." The action may vary in intensity according to the stimulus or internal state, but the basic pattern remains the same. These and other scientists were thus able to show that it is the brain and not the individual body part that "feels" sensation, but they were unable to explain how different regions in the brain and body communicated this information.

It was the Spanish histologist Santiago Ramòn y Cajal (1843-1926) who pieced together a vital missing link when he proposed the neuron theory and the law of dynamic polarization. Cajal traced the nerves from the sensory organs such as the eye to the brain and found that the sensory nerves project inward from peripheral dendrites and axons toward the brain. The motor nerves operate in reverse; the dendrites of the motor nerves are in the brain and spinal cord with axons projecting outwards toward the muscles. However, the question remained, how do impulses pass from one neuron to another? The neuron theory stated that every nerve cell branches and each branch meets at a junction. Sherrington was later to name these junctions "synapses," although the question of how impulses passed across these gaps remained unanswered until 1914 when Henry Hallett Dale isolated a compound called acetylcholine found in the ergot fungus. Dale found that when this substance was applied to a nerve ending it produced a response in the muscle. A further series of experiments by Dale together with the work of Loewi suggested that acetycholine was secreted by motor nerves in response to electrical stimulation and that acetycholine was the chemical agent by which nerves worked on muscles. It was the first neurotransmitter to be identified.

Charles Sherrington (1857-1952) carried out a series of animal experiments in which he separated and identified nerves leading to and from the spinal cord and the brainstem. He then divided the brainstem and spinal cord from higher regions in the brain and undertook further experiments to see what happened to these "brainless" creatures when the central nervous system acted without the executive control of higher regions of the brain. It was through this process that he was able to establish the existence of the reflex arc—the path along which sensory signals are gathered together and passed through the central nervous system, which reacts by turning specific groups of muscles on and off. He also realized that reflexes do not act in isolation; rather they act together in a coordinated system (of systems). The detailed findings of this work were published in "The Integrative Action of The Nervous System" (1906).

Thus, it was through the work of a number of scientists over many years that the beginnings of our modern understanding of reflexes and of the central nervous system was born. Subsequently reflexes have been chronicled by many authors for diagnostic, functional and developmental purposes.

It is now recognized that certain reflex reactions provide outward signs of level of functioning within the central nervous system. They can be used as tools to assess damage, disease and dysfunction within the central nervous system. The cardinal feature of a reflex is that the basic pattern of response remains unchanged and once initiated, the action

Neurons — individual cells that are the smallest unit of the nervous system.

Dendrites — short fibers that branch out from the cell body and pick up incoming messages.

Axon — the extension of a nerve cell along which impulses travel away from the cell body.

Neurotransmitter — a substance released from the axon terminal of a presynaptic neuron on excitation which diffuses across the synaptic cleft to excite or inhibit the target cell.

cannot be modified. This final observation provides the reason why there is such a profound impact upon the functioning and adaptability of the individual who is the servant rather than the master of his/her reflexes.

The model for assessment and remediation of reflexes in the context of learning and emotional problems outlined in the previous chapters started its journey to its present form from a number of sources. No history can ever paint a true picture of the past, because ideas are not born from a neat sequence of events but rather from knowledge and multiple influences collected over a long period of time. "The real history is the story of the struggle—the searchings, successes and failures as well as the personal interactions of everyone in the field." (Keeling 2001) Nevertheless, the system used by The Institute for Neuro-Physiological Psychology today emerged as a direct result of several key influences and authors:

One such author was A.E. Tansley who wrote the book, "Reading and Remedial Reading" (1967). One of Tansley's messages was this: just because a child looks normal, do not assume that he or she has the equipment to function well in the classroom. Tansley also introduced his readers to the work of the American educational psychologist Carl Delacato. In his book, "The Diagnosis and Treatment of Speech and Reading Problems" (1963). Delacato described how none of the children he had assessed with specific learning difficulties had been through the developmental motor stages of crawling on the stomach or creeping on hands and knees. He also observed that all of the learning impaired group had failed to achieve full one-sidedness and were therefore cross-lateral or ambilateral. Peter Blythe, then a Senior Lecturer in Applied Psychology (Education) at a Teacher's Training College in the north of England, presented these concepts to a group of his students. One of the students, David McGlown, asked if they could put together a test battery which he could use to test all children in a remedial class. It was to ascertain, among other things, whether they had the motor-developmental skills to crawl on the stomach and creep on hands and knees. The rationale behind this test procedure was, if they did not have the neuro-motor skills to crawl and creep when they were babies, they would not have these skills as older children unless they had been specifically trained. Blythe and McGlown also decided that the test battery should include tests for visual-perceptual functioning and visual-motor integration abilities, to ascertain whether the children had developed the eye movement skills and hand-eye coordination skills necessary to cope in a classroom. Tests for laterality were included to see if they had developed one-sidedness (unilaterality). Emotional status was also evaluated.

Nine subsequent years of research by Blythe and McGlown revealed a cluster of Central Nervous System dysfunctions which would formerly have been consistent with a diagnosis of Minimal Brain Dysfunction (MBD). The group studied consisted of children with emotional and behavior problems and included adults suffering from psychoneurotic symptoms and syndromes. It particularly included those whose problems had not yielded to what was then considered the therapy of choice. What was exciting was that the effect of the underlying dysfunction identified by Blythe and McGlown was not only measurable but could be remedied.

MBD has often been categorized with the term "maturational lag." Whatever term used, it must be compensated for in other ways. The law of compensation, however, exacts a price in other areas, and the price is often paid at the level of emotional functioning. Le Winn (1969) wrote that, "the effect of neurological impairment upon the individual is to place them in a chronic state of internal excitation whereby they will react to normally non-noxious stimuli." Clements (1966) had described children with a Minimal Brain Dysfunction as "children of near average, average or above average intelligence with certain learning or behavioral difficulties ranging from mild to severe, which are associated with deviations of function of the central nervous system. These deviations may manifest themselves in several combinations of impairment in perception, conceptualization of language, memory and control of attention, impulse or motor function." Wender (1971) listed some of the effects of MBD within the syndrome as including, "poor impulse control, anti-social behavior and impaired sphincter control" (some of the factors included in the category of Asperger's Syndrome today). He went on to describe how in interpersonal relationships "they are often obstinate, stubborn, negativistic, bossy, disobedient, sassy and impervious . . . they show four major types of dysfunction: increased lability, altered reactivity, increased aggressiveness and dysphoria" (many of the features of today's child given a diagnosis of Attention Deficit Hyperactive Disorder).

Within the category of Minimal Brain Dysfunction Clements had listed over 99 possible signs and symptoms of which 10 were the most salient. Such a vast collection of possible symptoms meant that almost anyone could at one time or another fit into the diagnostic term. This, together with the fact that "minimal" suggests the least possible, whereas the effects of Minimal Brain Dysfunction on the individual can be anything but minimal (Hagberg 1975), led the Scottish Child Neurologist, Tom Ingram (1973) to say that "Minimal Brain Dysfunction is not a diagnosis — it is an escape from making one."

Blythe and McGlown (1979) suggested that such terms as cortical immaturity, developmental cerebral deficit and developmental lag together with Minimal Brain Dysfunction could be described more precisely as **Organic Brain Dysfunction (OBD)**, which describes neurological impairment that has a functional organic basis and which is open to effective remedial intervention. It was the possibility of effective remedial intervention through the use of a specific physical program which heralded a major departure from previous diagnostic labels.

Organic Brain Dysfunction (OBD) was defined by Blythe and McGlown as the presence of three combined factors:

1. Affected patterns of motor development.

Each of these problems can be linked to immature reflexes, inadequate cortical control and/or biochemical imbalance.

Dysphoria: an emotional state characterized by anxiety, depression and restlessness or general malaise.

2. Evidence of cross-laterality or marked ambiguity of laterality above eight years of age.
3. Definite perceptual problems, including difficulty in Visual-Motor Integration (VMI).

(Blythe, McGlown 1979)

Later, Blythe found that each of the items listed in the diagnosis of OBD were present together with a cluster of immature reflexes.

The term OBD has since been replaced by the term **Neuro-Developmental Delay** that describes *measurable* immaturity in the functioning of the central nervous system as confirmed by a *cluster* of abnormal primitive and postural reflexes in an individual above three and a half years of age. Such a cluster of *abnormal reflexes* is accompanied by problems with control of *automatic balance, coordination, oculo-motor functioning* and *visual-perceptual difficulties*. Additional signs may include cross laterality or ambiguity of laterality, and problems with the processing of auditory information such as auditory delay and auditory confusion although such auditory problems can exist as a discrete category.

The term Neuro-Developmental Therapy was also used by physio-therapists trained in the Bobath techniques. The Bobath method was designed for use with children with Cerebral Palsy. In order to differentiate the two, INPP's method of intervention should carry the distinction NDT (INPP).

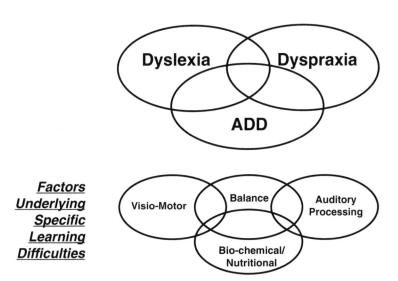

Factors Underlying Specific Learning Difficulties

Many of the signs and symptoms of NDD also overlap the diagnostic categories of Dyslexia, Dyspraxia, Attention Deficit Disorder (ADD) and Dysfunction of Attention, Motor, Perception (DAMP). We know that up to 80% of children diagnosed with Dyslexia have some symptoms of Dyspraxia and that up to 80% of children given a diagnosis of Dyspraxia in turn experience some problems in common with Dyslexia (difficulties with balance, orientation and motor skills). Both groups also share some problems with focusing and sustaining attention on specific tasks. Where these problems overlap, NDD is often a common underlying factor. Similarly adults with Agoraphobia and Panic Disorder tend to have deficits in the functioning of the vestibular apparatus and its connections to other parts of the central nervous system.

A summary of techniques used to remediate abnormal reflexes would be incomplete without mention of the earlier work of Temple Fay, Carl Delacato, Glenn Doman, and of others such as A. Jean Ayres and Florence Scott. Temple Fay, a neurosurgeon, developed a system of remediation for brain injury based on the knowledge of neurological organization. He developed a patterning treatment that was aimed directly at the injured brain rather than at the body part affected by that injury. Current thinking at that time viewed the cortex as the master controller of all brain and body functions. Fay proposed an opposite interpretation. He had come *". . . to view the brain organ (cortex) as the **child** of the spinal cord, developing through an evolutionary period extending over 600,000,000 years of vertebrate elaboration, and not the spinal cord as just the loyal servant and messenger of a capricious brain master."* In other words, he suggested that lower regions of the brain can be utilized to entrain the cerebral cortex and that remediation of injury in higher centers in the brain should use that knowledge — that not only does the higher brain control the body, but that the body can train the brain.

The word "remediate" is derived from the Latin "remedium" or medicine which has come to mean "something that corrects a wrong."

Motor training programs have been around for many years (Kephart, Cratty, Frostig, Lefroy, Kiphard). Many start at the crawling and creeping stages of development. The difference between reflex stimulation/inhibition programs and more general motor training programs is that the reflex program uses the ***reflexes*** as indicators of stages when development may have been temporarily arrested or omitted. The child who has retained early reflexes proceeds to the next developmental skill apparently without ill effect. Subtle gaps, however, remain in the "wiring" of the central nervous system as a result of the by-passed stage of development because learning normally experienced during the missed stage did not occur.

"Individuals still under the influence of early reflexes do not lack power; they lack control and proper release of power. The greater the primitive power, the less the skill (and control) of power." (Fay 1958)

A reflex stimulation/inhibition program aims to give the brain a "second chance" to experience the movements that should have been made in the early months of development. It thereby creates a bridge between the gaps and facilitates more efficient transmission and execution of messages passing between the brain and the body. Whereas many other methods of intervention work from the cortex *down* towards the brain stem, reflex stimulation and inhibition programs start from the spinal cord and brain stem and work *up* towards the cortex to access improved cortical control by providing more efficient pathways.

124

Clinical Research

Research into the area of reflexes has been carried out by many scientists in the fields of medicine, education and allied professions. A summary of some of the research over the last 30 years into the impact of abnormal reflexes on education and behavior might be of interest:

- In 1970, Gustafsson, an Occupational Therapist, carried out a study in which she compared the reflex levels of two groups of children: one group had been identified as having neurological impairment, the other group had no known neurological impairment. Reflex testing revealed a profile of abnormal reflexes in all of the group with neurological impairment. Eight out of the "normal" group which comprised a total of 19 children also had some reflex abnormalities. Of these eight, it was subsequently found that one had behavior problems and the remainder had either reading or writing problems.

- In 1971, Barbara Rider, an associate professor at the University of Kansas, who also was an Occupational Therapist, carried out a study in which she set out to assess the incidence of abnormal reflex responses in two groups of second grade children: Group 1 had learning disabilities; Group 2 had no identified learning problems. She found significantly more abnormal reflexes in the learning disabled group than the normal group. She then compared scores on the Wide Range Achievement Tests (WRAT) to see if there was a correlation with a child's abnormal reflex responses. Children whose reflexes fell within the normal range scored consistently higher on the WRAT tests than those who had abnormal reflexes.

- In the early 1970s at the University of Purdue, Dr. Miriam Bender examined the effect of just one reflex, the Symmetrical Tonic Neck Reflex (STNR) on education. She found the STNR to be present in 75% of a group of children with learning disabilities but not present in *any* of the children without a history of learning disabilities. She then went on to develop a series of exercises designed to help inhibit the STNR and found that many of the children improved as the STNR declined. This was later published as The Bender-Purdue Reflex Test (1976).

- In 1994, at the University of Newcastle-upon-Tyne, Wilkinson, a former student at INPP, carried out a replica study of Rider's 1971 research. Wilkinson also found a link between abnormal primitive reflexes and learning disability. She was also able to detect underachievement from the reflex profile. Detailed analysis of her results suggested that a retained Tonic Labyrinthine Reflex was a central factor. There also seemed to be a relationship between a retained Moro reflex and specific problems with mathmatical skills.

- In 1997, O'Dell and Cook, who had founded the Bender Institute in Indianapolis, found that Miriam Bender's exercises to inhibit the Symmetrical Tonic Neck Reflex were of value in overcoming hyperactivity.

- In 1998, Goddard and Hyland reviewed the validity of the developmental screening questionnaire devised by Blythe and McGlown (1979) when used as an initial screening device to identify individuals whose problems might have a neuro-developmental basis. Questions relating to 23 generally accepted milestones of early child development were given to parents of two groups of children. Answers were then analyzed and compared. Group 1 had a history of reading, writing and copying problems. Group 2 had no such difficulties. Statistical analysis revealed that a child with a score of 7 or more failures to have met these milestones belonged to the group with specific learning difficulties. Children scoring less than 2 did not. A score of 7 or more out of 23 was therefore necessary to identify a neuro-developmentally caused learning difficulty.

The two populations were also compared on individual questions to identify which early developmental factors were significant in predicting later learning difficulties. The criteria that revealed a marked difference between the two groups could be divided into two main categories:

1. Factors that relate to motor development and vestibular functioning:
   - Late at learning to walk (16 months or later)
   - Omission of the developmental stages of crawling and creeping
   - Difficulty dressing above 7 years of age (fine muscle coordination)
   - Difficulty learning to ride a bicycle above 7 years of age
   - Difficulty catching a ball
   - Difficulty sitting still
   - Bedwetting above the age of 5 years
2. Factors that relate to the development of phonological skills:
   - Late at learning to talk
   - History of frequent ear, nose and throat infections
   - Hypersensitive/overreacts to sound

Delays in both motor development and/or auditory processing can affect subsequent language-based skills.

No *single* criteria should be considered indicative of underlying neuro-developmental delay; rather *a profile of 7 or more factors* would suggest that further investigation is indicated. Table II (p.116) lists some of the developmental "markers" included in the questionnaire.

- In 2001, Goddard presented the results of Neuro-Developmental assessment on a sample of 54 children with Dyslexia.

  A sample of 54 children who had previously received an independent diagnosis of Dyslexia were examined for the presence of abnormal primitive and postural reflexes, cerebellar involvement, dysdiadochokinesia, oculo-motor dysfunction and visual-perceptual problems. The findings revealed that 100% of the sample showed evidence of a retained Asymmetrical Tonic Neck Reflex and a Tonic Labyrinthine Reflex. Other residual primitive reflexes of significance were: The Moro reflex (81%), the Symmetrical Tonic Neck Reflex (72%), the Spinal Galant reflex (65%) and the Palmar reflex (55%).

In addition, postural reflexes were shown to be **under-developed:**

Segmental Rolling Reflexes (90%)
Labyrinthine Headrighting Reflexes (88%) *vestibular*
Oculo-Headrighting Reflexes (87%) *visual*
Amphibian Reflex (74%)

53% of the sample showed some evidence of cerebellar involvement and 85% had difficulty with one of the tests for dysdiadochokinesia.

92% showed evidence of oculo-motor dysfunction of which the most significant was difficulty with hand-eye tracking (essential for writing). All of the sample had difficulty with one or several of the visual-perceptual tests.

Although no comparison group was used in this study, the high incidence of accepted signs of neurological dysfunction in the sample suggests that neurological dysfunction did play a significant part in the previously identified symptoms of Dyslexia. Abnormalities in early patterns of motor development do affect the acquisition of higher, more complex skills. As these then never become automatic, they can interfere with a child's ability to express intelligence through written language and motor dependent tasks.

Research into the impact of Reflex Stimulation/Inhibition programs

- **1982** The Dala Clinic Report published the results of a small study of 15 children in Gothenburg, Sweden, who had failed to respond to previous standard remedial intervention. All were given reflex stimulation/inhibition exercises. Five children failed to complete the program. Of the ten children who followed the program to the end, not one was any longer classified as having specific learning disabilities. There were also additional improvements. Those children who had been unable to swim had learned to swim, and those children who had formerly suffered from regular, severe headaches, no longer had headaches. (Bernhardsson and Davidson)

- **1988** Faulkner presented the findings of a small study carried out in a Buckinghamshire school in the United Kingdom. She took a group of children who had reading difficulties and divided them into three groups: Groups a) and b) had reading difficulties. Group c) were normal readers.

  Over a three month period the following intervention was given.
  a)   Received conventional remedial help on five days of the week for three months
  b)   Received no other remedial help but went on a reflex inhibition program four days of the week for three months
  c)   Received no intervention
  At the end of the three months, a final reading test was given.
  a)   Had improved by five months
  b)   Had improved by nine months
  c)   Had improved by three months and two weeks

- **2000** McPhillips, Hepper and Mulhern assessed the efficacy of an intervention program based on replicating the movements generated by the primary-reflex system during fetal and neonatal life. They assigned a group of children who had both a persistent Asymmetrical Tonic Neck Reflex and a poor standard of reading to three treatment groups:
  a)   experimental group (children were given a specific movement sequence)
  b)   placebo control (children were given non-specific movements)
  c)   control (no movements given)

The experimental group a) showed a significant decrease in the level of persistent reflex over the course of the study whereas the changes in the placebo and control groups were not significant. Retesting of reading ability using the Neale analysis showed that all groups had improved over time but the greatest improvement occurred in the experimental group. Writing speed also improved in the experimental group. (The movements used with the experimental group were based upon the reflex stimulation/inhibition movements originally devised at INPP.)

Martin McPhillips originally trained at The Institute for Neuro-Physiological Psychology, Chester, in the theory and administration of the diagnostic assessment procedures and application of reflex stimulation and inhibition exercises in 1989/90. He subsequently went on to do research in this area independently and carried out a separate study.

- **2001** Bein-Wierzbinski, a former post graduate student at INPP, presented the findings of a study of 52 elementary school children in Germany. She had investigated whether disturbances in oculo-motor function and visual perception could be corrected by means of an appropriate motor training program which focused on early motor development and primitive reflexes. All of the children were examined for abnormal reflexes, and eye movements were assessed using an infra-red computerized eye tracking machine. One half of the children who had abnormal reflexes were given a reflex stimulation/inhibition program. The other half were examined both at the beginning and the end of the program but were not included in any training. A further six children who had reading and writing problems but no abnormal reflexes were also assessed at the beginning and the conclusion of the study to document any developmental improvements which might have occurred normally during the intervening time.

She found improvement in oculo-motor functioning and reading skills as persistent reflexes were corrected. Oculo-motor defects continued to persist in the control group who had not received specific motor training exercises.

- **2000/2001** Cherqui undertook a small double blind study in which she investigated whether cranio-sacral osteopathic dysfunctions found at birth and still present in a group of older children had an effect upon delayed neuro-motor development (confirmed by the presence of a cluster of abnormal primitive and postural reflexes). A connection might be found if osteopathic treatment affected a modification of the neuro-motor responses.

Independent assessment of the reflexes was carried out before and after 3 sessions of cranio-osteopathic intervention, which were carried out at two-week intervals over a period of 6 weeks. At the first assessment the presence of a cluster of abnormal reflexes showed that the central nervous system of these children was not supported by a firm integration of the different stages of neurological development.

The osteopathic intervention, by reestablishing the mobility of the cranio-sacral structure and by stopping irritation and subsequent excitability which resulted from osteopathic lesions, reactivated the hierarchic progression of the reflexes. Reassessment of the reflexes at the conclusion of the treatment revealed increased inhibition of the primitive reflexes, but some regression in the profile of the postural reflexes. This suggested that the osteopathic intervention may have started a reorganization of postural tonicity in a cephalo-caudal sequence in line with the passage of normal development. This reorganization allowed the children to reassert different stages of the tonicity of the medial axis (related to the cranio-sacral axis) and the balance between flexor and extensor tone. *Comment: Caution should be exercised in the interpretation of these results because the intervention was only carried out over a relatively short period of time and did not take into account either possible re-emergence of the primitive reflexes at a later stage or, indeed, later improvement.* **Any re-emergence of the primitive reflexes following the correction of an osteopathic lesion would be a clear indication that remedial intervention should be complemented by a reflex stimulation/inhibition program.** The initial findings, however, are of interest, and appear to suggest that the reflexes respond to a number of different treatment modalities and there is definite room for further research and longitudinal studies in the areas of osteopathic application.

SUMMARY

The presence of a primitive or lack of a postural reflex at key stages in development may be seen as evidence of continuing subcortical control over neuromuscular functions. Voluntary control of movements directly reflects the degree of cortical control in the individual — the cortex represents purposive behavior whereas subcortical behavior is limited and stereotyped. Subcortical systems may remain dominant for a variety of reasons: lack of use at an early stage in development; lack of inhibition; metabolic or pathological conditions or, possibly, directly through injury. Retained primitive reflexes are a symptom of incomplete cortical inhibition. Damage or dysfunction higher in the brain may release them from cortical control, or the retention of reflexes may in itself interfere with the establishment of full cortical control. Detection and analysis of primitive and postural reflexes can therefore be used as a valuable tool in assessing the level of remediation required by a child. It indicates the developmental stage a child has reached. Being able to pinpoint this exact stage also helps to determine the teaching method from which a child is likely to benefit most.

The reflexes, however, provide only the substrata for later learning, and by the time a child has reached the age of 8 years, other systems will also have become involved. The reflexes are only one sign of misdirection in development, which may then be accompanied by dysfunctions in the processing of auditory information, visual information, vestibular functioning etc.

It is therefore important to unravel which area presents the greatest stumbling block for the individual child and to devise a personalized program. For, although the symptoms of dysfunction may be similar for many children, the developmental route the child has had to take to compensate for his problems is as individual as he is. This is why a battery of tests can be invaluable in assessing the needs of the individual child.

The key areas for investigation should include tests for:
- Balance
- Gross muscle coordination
- Fine muscle coordination
- Cerebellar functioning
- Primitive and Postural Reflexes
- Laterality
- Oculo-motor Functioning
- Visual-Perceptual performance
- Auditory discrimination and auditory laterality
- Performance on specific age related tasks

To complicate the search for answers, there is also the possibility that other factors may be part of the overall problem: poor nutrition is one. In our affluent Western world a surfeit of junk food can result in a profile of vitamin and mineral depletion which constitutes a new form of malnutrition. Allergies, detrimental social environment, emotional insecurity, genetic or biochemical influences and psychological problems may also contribute.

A neuro-developmental approach enables the teacher/therapist/clinician to "take the lid off learning difficulties" to see what lies beneath. It allows them to look again at the question posed by A.E. Tansley over 20 years ago: *For far too long teachers have concentrated upon the psychological problems of the child, or the socio-economic environment, instead of asking the question, does the child have the equipment which he needs to succeed at the educational level asked of him and the methods imposed on him?*

It was this question which first led Peter Blythe into the search for a physical basis for learning disabilities. The methods developed by Peter Blythe and David McGlown were then taken to Sweden by Catharina Johannesson Alvegård in the 1970s, to the United States in the 1980s, Germany and Ireland in the 1990s, and are now incorporated into many teachers' "thinking" throughout the world: If the foundations upon which learning is built are made strong, then teaching methods can become effective and the child can start to grow. In our modern world there is little room for academic failure, and if it seems to exist we must continue to ask the question WHY? Only when we start to understand why, can we begin to offer effective help in overcoming difficulties.

Appendix 1

Chapter Notes

Chapter 2 — Note 1

Investigation of postural reflex mechanisms began as early as 1824 when Flourens noted the disturbances of movement and posture that occurred in a pigeon when its vestibular canals were destroyed. Postural reflexes might better be described as movement reflexes. They are those reflexes that provide the basis for the development of voluntary movements and adaptive responses which should be available at a sub-cortical (subconscious) level to be called upon at any time in response to environmental change.

Chapter 2 — Note 2

Sometimes a subject will present a profile where the primitive reflexes are inhibited but the postural reflexes are underdeveloped. These children appear to compensate well and may not be identified as having problems until relatively late in development — sometimes well into adolescence or beyond. Paradoxically, these are the children who would have benefited from a motor training or sensory integration program at an earlier age. The specific problems this group show are typically problems in: adaptation, applying known concepts (problem solving), linking, multi-processing, sequencing and coping with large volumes of information — all skills which become essential at higher levels of education (secondary level and beyond).

Additional related problems in adolescents and young adults may include: a history of fine motor disturbances, low energy levels which mimic depression but do not respond to medication, lack of torso flexibility and difficulty carrying out complex movement patterns such as those required for martial arts and dance routines. Often the individual will comment on having to "think through" each movement sequence and having difficulty adapting to rapid changes in routine. (Beuret 2000)

The effect of under-developed postural reflexes is rather like having a limited environmental and social vocabulary. The individual can cope as long as the rules remain the same and they can continue to utilize a learned skill. If the rules required by a situation change, they need to "learn and practice" the new rules rather than being able to adapt and change to meet the altered circumstances. This can result in "awkwardness," feelings of personal and social inadequacy and increased propensity to suffer from anxiety.

Chapter 3 — Note 1

For over a century the cerebellum has been seen as a motor organ. A growing body of research now suggests that the cerebellum is involved in far more than the regulation of various aspects of motor learning. Studies of patients with cerebellar atrophy imply that it also plays a part in visuo-motor learning and adaptation, planning, strategic thinking, time processing (Ivry and Keele 1989) and associative learning. Further evidence from studies which have used functional imaging (PET and MRI) support the hypothesis that the cerebellum acts in concert with other structures as part of a frontal-subcortical system devoted to the storage and organization of timed sequential behaviors (Hallett and Grafman 1997), associative learning (Leiner, Leiner and Dow 1986, 1993), word generation (Posner and Raichle 1994) and rapid shifting of attention from one task to another. (Courchesne et al. 1994)

Some studies have found the cerebellum of certain autistic children to be smaller than normal and it has been suggested that this may lie behind the autistic child's tendency to become fixated on certain stereotyped activities and inability to shift attention to appropriate external stimuli. Another interpretation is that the autistic child has inadequate filtering mechanisms for shutting out unwanted sensory stimuli, is overloaded by too much sensory information and that repetitive stereotyped activities are a way of shutting out the external world, focusing on an inner world which may not be unlike a dream state, thereby reducing the anxiety produced by sensory overload.

Nicolson and Fawcett (1994, 1995) concluded that the cerebellum appears to be involved in the automization of basic skills related to motor competency, phonological processing and visual preception — skills found to be deficient in individuals diagnosed with Dyslexia. These are problems which are also present in children who have a cluster of abnormal primitive and postural reflexes.

Chapter 3 — Note 2

Leiner et al (1986) have argued that it is the unique enlargement of the neodentate in man that has enabled him to improve the performance of any other part of the brain to which it is linked as a result of two-way neural connections.

Chapter 3 — Note 3

Hallett and Grafman (1997) suggest that, "the role of the cerebellum in timed sequential cognitive processing may be analogous to its role in motor processing and suggest a mechanism by which cognitive events become sequenced and temporally labeled."

Chapter 3 — Note 4

As early as 1944 Snider and Stowell found that the tactile, visual and auditory centers of the cerebellum are linked to corresponding areas in the cerebral cortex. This led Snider to conclude that, *"the cerebellum is equally involved in the coordination of touch, hearing and sight as it is with movement . . . it is an accessory control system imposed upon the basic ascending (sensory) and descending (motor) circuits of the motor system."* This observation opens up many possibilities for remedial intervention.

Levinson uses anti-motion sickness and anti-histamine medication which have a direct effect upon the functioning of the vestibular-cerebellar circuit and connections to the reticular activating system. Levinson (1991) described children with vestibular-cerebellar problems as "upside-down kids" because their perceptual and metabolic systems react to certain types of medication in reverse. Not only do they produce cognitive evidence of directional confusion such as letter and word reversal when writing and spelling, but many of them are hypersensitive to specific medication sometimes responding to tranquilizing drugs with hyperactivity and becoming sedated after administration of stimulants. By fine-tuning the operation of these circuits, he claims to have evidence of alteration in cognitive functioning and behavior.

Chapter 3 — Note 5

Steffert (1997) suggested that there may be two distinct types of learners: "sign minds and design minds." She found that among a group of art and design students, many had a history of difficulty with *written* expression. They had found it easier to express themselves through pictorial or three-dimensional mediums and they had struggled with essay writing. It was her contention that they may have had undiagnosed features of Dyslexia. On the other hand, Portwood (2001) stated that Dyspraxia is *right* hemisphere dysfunction involving difficulty with spatial skills and the ability to visualize, ideate and execute controlled voluntary movement.

Chapter 3 — Note 6

The stages of his brain growth and the movements he makes are inextricably linked. Continuous brain development is facilitated through these movement sequences which lay down efficient neural pathways. *"Practice and repetition of movement patterns result in them being absorbed into the individual's repertoire of skills, probably also resulting in physical changes taking place in the neurons concerned, so that the flow of impulses along a specific pathway is facilitated. Repetition enhances facilitation and adeptness."* (Draper 1993)

Chapter 4 — Note 1

During the course of evolution, this region has become more complex in mammals and has developed into the labyrinthine *portion of the inner ear that houses the organs of balance and of hearing.* In embryonic development the upper portion of the labyrinth forms three hollow semicircular tubes each arranged at right angles to each other which will eventually form the basis for the control of balance. After birth it can detect movements of the head from the motion of the fluid inside these three small tubes. Each tube responds to motion in a different plane in relation to gravity.

The lower half of the labyrinth stretches into a long tube which coils to form a shell-like structure. The is the cochlea, the hearing apparatus which functions by detecting sound vibrations. Both organs together with the jaw, facial muscles, swallow mechanism and organs of speech production are evolutionary developments from the gill bars of our fish ancestors. The lateral line receptor has also formed projections to the brainstem which represent the structural foundation for the cerebellum (Larsell 1947). The cerebellum of higher species plays a dominant role in sensory-motor integration and coordination but is heavily dependent upon reciprocal interaction with vestibular centers.

Chapter 4 — Note 2

DeKlein (1924) and Magnus (1924) believed that functionally, the vestibular system is inseparable from the proprioceptive, visual and motor systems in the acquisition of developmental reflexes and of postural control. Together with the cerebellum it is involved in the maintenance of equilibrium, direction of eye gaze and the maintenance of a plane of vision dependent upon head position. These functions are achieved as a result of modification by the vestibular system of underlying muscle tone and neuromuscular reflexes. Mismatch between the vestibular, visual and proprioceptive systems can result in sensations of vertigo, motion sickness and anxiety.

Vestibular control underpins balance, poise and according to Hubbard (1971) provides the foundation for "the relationship of body image and motion which endlessly reflects changes in the social, moral, professional and personal life of an individual." It was Paul Schilder's (1993) belief that "organic changes in the vestibular apparatus might be highly significant in the etiology of certain neuroses and psychoses," a concept later followed up by Levinson and Blythe and McGlown (1979), Blythe (1990). While Levinson treated the symptoms of vestibular-cerebellar dysfunction with anti-motion sickness medication, Blythe went on to develop vestibular and reflex inhibition programs to treat the symptoms of Agoraphobia and Panic Disorder in adults all of whom he had found to have problems with balance and immaturity in the functioning of the central nervous system.

Chapter 4 — Note 3

Adequate vestibular input is essential for the automatic control of balance, posture and controlled voluntary action. Shaskan and Roller (1985) suggest that "a newborn's body tone, its fear of falling, the Moro reflex and the neck-righting reflex may all be expressions of the sequential development of the central nervous system and its relative normalcy or pathology."

Chapter 4 — Note 4

The relationship between the vestibular, visual and somatosensory systems and the link to arousal and attention is beautifully described by Allan Hobson in "The Dreaming Brain" . . .

"The intermediate brainstem serves not only as a way station for reflex information from spinal cord to cortex (and vice versa) but as a mode selector for both structures determining the ratio of stimulated to spontaneous neuronal information processing.

In evolution, the brainstem was one of the first structures to be added to the purely segmental spinal cord. In many primitive animals, the brainstem was all there was. It enabled organisms to achieve control of such special sense organs as eyes and to coordinate the increasing number of motor acts that developed as animals became more specialized with respect to limb functions. Thus, the brainstem contains within it the neurons that move the eyes and neurons capable of coordinating those eye movements with the position of the head and the body. The complex orchestration of head, eye and body position is conducted by the oculo-motor, reticular and vestibular systems of the brain."

Chapter 4 — Note 5

Attention and arousal demand precise control of eye and head position . . .

"Lorento de No (1933) showed that every change in head position is immediately and accurately translated by the vestibular system into an appropriate change in eye position. Also participating in this neuronal calculation are the cerebellum and the reticular formation. We know that Lorento de No's circuit is spontaneously activated in rapid eye movement (REM) or dreaming sleep so that head, eye and body position signals are internally generated. Thus when lying immobile in bed one has dream sensations of running, turning, and even flying."

Chapter 4 — Note 6

Most of a child's early touch experiences are provided by the mother during the feeding, changing and play. Allan Schore (1994) suggests that the mother acts as the primary facilitator in the early months for the formation of connections between different levels in the brain and the laying of foundations not only for later learning ability but also for emotional functioning and immune response. *"By providing well modulated socioaffective stimulation, the mother facilitates the growth of connections between cortical, limbic and subcortical limbic structures that neurobiologically mediate self-regulatory functions . . . the core of the self lies in patterns of affect regulation that integrate a sense of the self, lies in patterns of affect regulation that integrate a sense of self across state transitions, thereby allowing for a continuity of inner experience."*

Early handling is an important part of this process. Diamond et al (1963) describe the mother as "playing the role of higher brain structures: she is the child's auxilliary cortex."

Appendix 2

Case Studies and Selected Papers

(By permission of Dr. Lawrence Beuret, M.D., Chicago)

CASE 1: Adolescent 1

Adolescent 1 was referred for evaluation for possible Neuro-Development Delay because of unusual scatter in scores on the WISC-III *(Weschler Intelligence Scale for Children).*

He was 16 years of age. He had no history of any difficulty in learning to read but he had never shown any interest in reading outside of school. There was no sign of visual disturbances such as skipping of lines when reading, but he complained of headaches and concentration drifting after 15-30 minutes of reading.

He was not aware of specific writing difficulties, but he had not made the complete transition from printing to cursive writing. At the time of first assessment he ranked 17th from the bottom of a class of 675.

Neuro-Development assessment revealed lack of Headrighting Reflexes. Amphibian and Segmental Rolling Reflexes were slightly underdeveloped and there were traces of an Asymmetrical Tonic Neck Reflex, Tonic Labyrinthine Reflex and Moro Reflex still present, but the primitive reflex scores were not sufficiently high to account for his presenting problems.

After 6 weeks on a reflex stimulation/inhibition program, it was reported that reading was easier, there was no sign of headache or eye strain and he was able to remember details of what he had read. Writing had changed entirely to cursive script and he was attaining a B grade average in three classes. He had also bought a book to read for pleasure.

CASE 2: Adolescent 2

Adolescent was 13 years of age at the time of assessment. His presenting symptom was difficulty with fine motor coordination.

At 5 years of age, testing had indicated that he might belong in the range of "gifted" children, but it was noted that his movements were very tense and he had difficulty getting written work done.

At 10 years of age he was not doing written assignments or keeping on task. By 11 years he was actively resisting writing anything down. At the time of assessment (13 years) he avoided writing, and if pressed, would run sentences together wihout punctuation or capital letters. When writing, he had to prop his head up with one hand. When assessed, he did not have the usual history consistent with writing problems, such as early fine motor difficulties, complaints of hand or arm pain with prolonged writing, or poor penmanship. His reflex profile showed only a minimal level of ATNR, certainly not consistent with the level of writing difficulty that he was experiencing. He did have underdeveloped headrighting reflexes, amphibian reflex and segmental rolling reflexes from the shoulders.

Two areas of his history raised the suspicion of inadequate postural reflex involvement:
1. The need to support his head when writing.
2. Running of sentences together without punctuation or capitalization.

Two months after starting a reflex stimulation/inhibition program, his mother reported that he was less resistant about writing and had begun to use capital letters and punctuation correctly. He was also sitting in a normal position to write.

CASE 3: Adult 1

Adult 1 was 30 years of age and had been referred for assessment by a psychiatrist for problems with attention. He had been prescribed Ritalin in the past but had not responded to it.

He had experienced reading problems since the first grade but was not considered learning disabled. He had received tutoring between the first and twelfth grades and had struggled through high school and college. Reading more than two pages resulted in fatigue, loss of focus, headache and eye irritation. Vision therapy had helped at 9 years of age but had not solved all of these problems. At the age of 30 his reading level was equivalent to sixth grade.

He did not suffer from motion sickness (a common indicator of underlying Neuro-Developmental problems in adolescents and adults if it persists beyond puberty), but he complained of difficulty focusing and keeping his place if he tried to read in a car.

Ritalin *(Methylphenidate)* is a stimulant drug (amphetamine group) used to treat Attention Deficit Disorder (ADD) and Attention Deficit Hyperactive Disorder (ADHD). The group of drugs to which Ritalin belongs affect synapses where norepinephrine and dopamine are transmitters. The primary known action is to increase the amount of neurotransmitter at the synapse by blocking reuptake, or in larger doses, to increase neurotransmitter release. It is still not known whether this is the mechanism through which Ritalin regulates hyperactivity. Another suggestion is that it helps to boost the firing rate of the Beta brain waves (the brain waves that should keep us in an alert waking state and which are thought to be underactive in ADHD), thereby enabling the patient to concentrate more easily without needing continuous activity. 1:4 cases do not respond to drug therapy.

When writing he often mixed printing and cursive script and prolonged writing resulted in word omissions and spelling errors.

By 14 years of age he was experimenting with drugs and at the time of assessment was enrolled in Alcoholics Anonymous.

His reflex profile showed minimal traces of primitive reflex activity. Oculo- and Labyrinthine Head Righting reflexes were underdeveloped, as were the Amphibian and Segmental Rolling reflexes. Testing for the Labyrinthine Head Righting reflexes had resulted in feelings of vertigo. In addition to a reflex assessment, he undertook the Minnesota Multiphasic Personality Inventory.

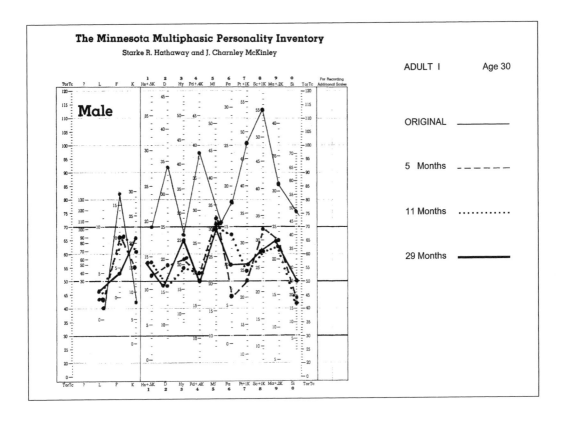

The Minnesota Multiphasic Personality Inventory
Starke R. Hathaway and J. Charnley McKinley

ADULT I   Age 30

Male

ORIGINAL _____

5 Months ------

11 Months ....

29 Months _____

The initial MMPI profile (solid line) showed significant elevations on the following scales:

1. Hypochondria —preoccupation with physical symptoms
2. **Depression**
3. Hysterical
4. **Anti-social behavior**
5. Identity
6. Paranoia (hypersensitivity to criticism)
7. **Anxiety**
8. **Disturbed memory and concentration**
9. **Impulsivity**
10. **Withdrawal from social contact**

(criteria in **bold** *= significant elevation at time of first assessment)*

Retesting at 5 and 11 months after the commencement of a reflex stimulation/inhibition program showed the profile to be within normal limits (dotted line).

Other changes of significance as treatment progressed were:
• Ability to read and focus for one hour or more.
• Improved ability to recognize unfamiliar words which would previously have been skipped over.
• Cessation of lower back tension.
• Improved organizational skills at work.
• Parents and AA sponsor both commented on increased energy and productivity.
• Golf improved.
• Used to watch only CNN and sports TV; now able to enjoy documentaries.
• Auditory processing improved.

After 30 weeks on the program, he was able to absorb more information from reading material the first time. He was studying for the stock broker's exam and doing well on practice tests.

SELECTED PAPERS by Sally Goddard

ELECTIVE MUTISM: THE UNCHOSEN SILENCE !

The term "selective mutism" formerly described as "elective mutism" infers a voluntary refusal to speak in certain situations. DSM IV (1995)—with a cross reference from ELECTIVE MUTISM—describes its characteristics as follows:

"The essential feature of selective mutism is the persistent failure to speak in specific social situations, (e.g. school, with playmates) where speaking is expected, despite speaking in other situations. (This diagnosis should not be given if it lasts for less than a month, the child has no knowledge of the subject being discussed, or suffers from other forms of language or developmental disorders, or schizophrenia.) Instead of communicating by standard verbalization, children with this disorder may communicate by gestures, nodding or shaking the head, or pulling or pushing, or in some cases by monosyllabic, short or monotone utterances, or in an altered voice."

"Associated features include: Excessive shyness, fear of social embarrassment, social isolation and withdrawal, clinging, compulsive traits, temper tantrums or other controlling or oppositional behavior, particularly in the home."

Selective/elective mutism is a separate condition from autism, but in certain circumstances it might be viewed as a minor form of autism or a manifestation of a particular autistic type of behavior. One autistic 17 year old who had been unable to talk since the age of 6, was later able to write down her experiences of being locked in the silent world. (Hocking. 1990)

(The following original text was written without punctuation of any kind. Minimal punctuation has been inserted by the writer to facilitate easier reading.)

"Caroline wanted to talk so much. but it seemed to be an impossible task. "Do you think she will ever talk?" was the question that everyone always asked her mother and her teacher, to which they replied. "There is no reason why she shouldn't. All the apparatus is there. She used to talk when she was a little girl."

Some people found this hard to believe. They thought her parents must be deluding themselves and that she had always been silent. But she had spoken. She could remembers quite clearly the times she had said things to her Mommy. "Look at the moon!" she said one day, caught by the sudden beauty of it in the daytime sky. She must have been about six years old at the time, lost in her misery, but still responsive to beauty coming unawares from the heavens. She could remember other times when she had tried to say things, but had been caught in the black web of her unhappiness and unable to utter a sound. It is very difficult to explain the way in which her fear gripped her vocal chords. It felt as though unseen hands were pressing on her throat struggling to extinguish life itself. Such a little place for the air to come and go, and so little room for the mysterious life force to exist. That area of her body seemed so especially vulnerable, so very exposed, that it must be protected at all costs, even the cost of silence. It seemed to save valuable air for the process of life itself. There was none to spare for eventual speech, so speech had to go. No one realized that this was one of the fears behind the silence: this sense of tight breathlessness that seemed to suffocate and threaten what little life there was with extinction. This was a real feeling when she was a tiny girl, but it was not until she was nearly grown up that she had the detachment to describe it. It was the same with so many feelings now that she was older. She could give a description to the things that had hurled great doubts and fears at her small mind. She had the words to describe what it had all been like that's why she felt it was so important to write a book to explain. As her teacher had said, she was in a position to help others. Real experience, ably described, was worth a ton of suppositions by wellmeaning experts. What hurt so much was the widely held belief that students of psychiatry seemed to hold: If you were silent you could not understand. If you didn't use language you couldn't express any thoughts. But how did they know that a lot of speechless people hadn't got heads full of beautiful expressive language that they couldn't use, because no one had found the key to their confidence."

It would be very easy to analyze this girl's feelings in terms of psychological etiology, but it is the purpose of this paper to argue that elective mutism has an underlying physical basis and to examine the underlying mechanisms which in certain situations might inhibit the organs of speech production.

Two of the most powerful images that this girl's description evokes are those of fear and of breathlessness. Many phrases in the English language imply a connection between fear and the inability to talk: "petrified," "speechless with fear," "frozen to the spot," "tongue tied" and "struck dumb"— each one a recognition of a normal, momentary response to extreme fear. The question that poses itself here is: Why should certain individuals experience such extreme fear in the course of their day-to-day living, even to the extent that they cannot operate or interact effectively with the outside world?

An explanation may be found within the concept of neuro-developmental delay (NDD). Neuro-developmental delay encompasses a variety of symptoms, of which elective mutism may be one. These symptoms emanate from an arrested or omitted stage of development during either the fetal or the infantile period. Subsequent development proceeds normally thereafter, but an underlying weakness or immaturity remains within the central nervous system (CNS) which may cause other systems in the body to misfire under certain conditions. The existence and extent of neuro-developmental delay is measured by the presence and the strength of primitive reflexes beyond the normal age of inhibition, and the absence of postural reflexes. The latter should have developed to allow the individual to manipulate and interact effectively within the environment. These aberrant reflexes provide signposts of central nervous system (CNS) maturity.

During normal development, the primitive reflexes should start to emerge, strengthen, fulfill a function, and then undergo inhibition throughout the first year of life. There should be a strict chronology, sequence, and rhythm to this reflex structure, so that by a certain age specific milestones should have been achieved. Should the sequence be interrupted in any way it will result in the early reflexes remaining locked in the system, so that the emergence of subsequent reflexes is disturbed, and further central nervous system development will be built upon eccentric foundations.

The earliest known reflexes to emerge are those that appear at 5-7 weeks after conception and which form a group of "withdrawal reflexes." These represent the earliest observed realization of tactile awareness in the embryo who, when barely visible to the naked eye, will respond to tactile stimulation in the mouth region with a rapid amebiclike withdrawal movement of the whole organism. It has been suggested (Goddard, 1989) that the early withdrawal reflex may be a manifestation of the fear paralysis reflex (FPR) described in detail by Kaada (1986), and which can have important implications in later life if it does not undergo inhibition during the gestational period.

Capute (1986) divides the primitive reflexes into three categories:
1.   Intrauterine reflexes that appear and are suppressed during intrauterine development, (not present at birth).
2.   Intrauterine/Birth reflexes
      Reflexes that appear during later intrauterine development, are present at birth. and are inhibited by 6 months of age.
3.   Postural reflexes
      Reflexes that appear during late infancy following inhibition of the primitive reflexes.

The withdrawal reflexes belong to the first category and should be inhibited at the time of the emergence of the Moro reflex at 9-32 weeks after conception. This suggests that the Moro reflex itself plays an inhibitory role for the preceding reflex, and it is only the development of a full and strong Moro reflex which will complete this task. If the Moro reflex fails to develop fully during this period, then both the withdrawal reflexes and the Moro reflex will remain "locked" and active in the system beyond the normal age of inhibition.

How can the presence of these two reflexes impair later functioning—and particularly the mechanisms of speech—if they remain active at the subcortical level beyond the age of inhibition?

Kaada (1986) described the characteristics of the fear paralysis reflex using the analogy of the "terrified rabbit," who becomes frozen to the spot at which he has first experienced sudden fear. In the animal kingdom it may serve a useful purpose where the motionless animal will not attract the attention of its predator. Within mankind, it represents a maladaptive response to situations with which the individual is unable to cope.

Its accompanying characteristics are also of significance: Activation of the fear paralysis reflex results in immediate motor paralysis accompanied by respiratory arrest in expiration. Muscle tone is reduced and there is lack of response to external stimuli. A pain suppressing mechanism is released, together with bradycardia and peripheral vasoconstriction. Kaada states that it is "a reflex present in the entire animal kingdom which is temporarily released from cortical control as a result of extreme fear." If it fails to undergo full inhibition at the correct time in humans. then it remains active at the subcortical level, lowering the threshold of fear in the individual, so that it can be activated by minor stimuli which present no actual threat to the individual at all.

The Moro reflex should emerge from 9-32 weeks after conception, be fully present at birth, and undergo inhibition at 3-4 months of neonate life. At 9-12 weeks other vital systems in the body are also developing: the vestibular system, the cerebellum and the hypothalamus. If the Moro reflex, which is the fetus' primitive alerting mechanism to stress or threat, does not develop fully at this time, it is possible that the fetus' stress responses may be inadequate. For example, (Odent 1986) describes how the entire hormonal profile for later life is regulated during this dynamic period of development.

"At an early stage of fetal life the pituitary gland, which controls all other endocrine glands, can secrete all the known pituitary hormones. When the fetus is 11-12 weeks old, the vessels that will become the hypothalamus and the pituitary glands come together. By that time. the hypothalamus is already controlling the pituitary. and by the time the fetus is 3 months old, the day-to-day variations in the stress hormone ACTH are already well established."

Specific hormonal states at an age when the basic adaptive system has not reached maturity may set the hormonal levels for life. For instance, if the fetus, or baby is in constant unalleviated stress, this will result in the release of stress hormones and regulate the hypothalamus in such a way, that the seeds for future conditions such as poor stress tolerance and hypertension are sown.

The hypothalamus acts as a bridge between the brain and the hormonal system —it belongs to both, and it plays a leading role in responses to psychological stress. Together with the limbic lobe it stimulates the pituitary axis, the reticular activating system and the sympathetic arm of the autonomic nervous system —three separate circuits that respond to unfamiliarities and to challenge. Activation of these three circuits leads to the release of the stress hormone ACTH together with other hormones from the brainstem and sympathetic nerves, which result in a rise in heart rate, dilation of the pupils, and increased discharge of the reticular activating system which in turn results in increase in muscle tension, rise in blood pressure and heart rate, and the inhibition of reflex bradycardia. These are all the physical symptoms of the activated Moro reflex, which has sometimes been referred to as the initiator of the "fight or flight" mechanism. The Moro may also be regarded as the "release" mechanism from an activated fear paralysis reflex.

What might be the result of both the fear paralysis reflex (FPR) and the Moro reflex remaining active at the subcortical level in an individual?

We would have a person with a low fear threshold and a low stress threshold. A person who may be hypersensitive to touch, sound, specific frequencies of sound, changes in his visual field, smell and possibly taste as well. He may be able to compensate and overcome his hypersensitivity in many situations, but it will involve conscious "over-riding" of instinctive reflexive responses by the cortex. He will become quickly fatigued, and with the fatigue his ability to compensate will be reduced, so that a reflexive response is more easily elicited. Which particular reflex is elicited will depend upon the circumstances. In certain situations both reflexes will be overcome by conscious control and the individual will react to that situation rationally and effectively. At other times, the situation might provoke the Moro or overreaction response. On another occasion the withdrawal reflexes will claim priority, and the individual will find it impossible to respond at all. Elective mutism may be the result of the latter.

What remains to be answered, however, is this: Why should specific social situations provoke such extreme fear?

Where the fear paralysis reflex (FPR) and the Moro Reflex remain, later reflexes in the hierarchical structure will also be aberrant to some degree. The tonic labyrinthine reflex (TLR) may remain in its residual or retained form, so that any movement of the head forwards or backwards beyond the midline point will result in automatic flexion or extension of the arms and the legs—a response that can only be controlled by conscious muscular effort. In that case, balance in the upright position will never be stable or constant. Furthermore, the labyrinthine and oculo-headrighting reflexes which should be present at 6 months of age will not develop fully. This in turn will affect oculomotor functioning.

The tonic labyrinthine reflex (TLR) also exerts a direct influence upon the labyrinth. The labyrinth is a complex organ for attaining balance, which, by movement of fluid in three orthogonal tubes operates rather like a spirit level (carpenter's level) activating special nerves which send signals to the brain concerning movement of the head. The vestibular apparatus then detects changes of direction and position of the head in space, particularly when the movement starts and stops. Information from the vestibular apparatus is combined with information from other sensory channels. Both prenatally and after birth, the vestibular system controls body image impression, and also kinesthesia (the sensation of bodily movement in space).

The vestibular apparatus is also a filtering point for sound. The ear acts as a collecting organ not only for sound stimuli, but also for those stimuli that are responsible for coordinating the vestibular portion of the labyrinth. (Tomatis, 1980) If, as a result of aberrant reflexes, the vestibular is dealing with conflicting messages from other sensory channels, it may impair its ability to process and relay sound messages to the language processing centers in the cortex. The addition of a tonic labyrinthine reflex (TLR) to a fear paralysis reflex (FPR) and a Moro reflex, imposes a new set of problems on the individual. Balance is rarely under automatic control, oculomotor functioning may be erratic and there may be severe sound discrimination problems, so that the individual suffers from the "cocktail party deafness" phenomenon. A string of words together may sound like a meaningless unit. Individual conversation within a group may be perceived as a conglomerate of jumbled sounds which do not immediately make sense. This condition is sometimes referred to as "auditory delay" or "auditory confusion". Such an individual may have a heightened sensitivity to certain frequencies of sound with a lowered sensitivity to other frequencies, with the result that parts of words are not easily registered, and miscellaneous sounds may intrude more readily on the listener's consciousness. Under these circumstances, the environment becomes a disorientating and bewildering one. Each one of us has known at sometime how unpleasant and frightening it is to he lost in a strange place. The child with a strong tonic labyrinthine reflex (TLR), Moro reflex and fear paralysis reflex (FPR), knows what it is like to be "lost" many times in each waking day. In such situations the FPR is easily elicited.

The vestibular apparatus is also linked to the vagus or the tenth cranial nerve at the level of the medulla. (Blythe, 1990) The vagus nerve contains both sensory and motor fibers. The sensory fibers convey sensitivity to part of the external ear, and carry afferent impulses from the pharynx and the larynx and the internal organs of the thorax and abdomen. The motor fibers and accessory nerves serve the striated muscles of the palate, the larynx and the pharynx. If a child is already overloaded by outside stimuli, his compensatory mechanisms are stretched to capacity, so that there is little energy available for expression. Far too much attention is concentrated upon making sense of conflicting perceptions. The confused vestibular excites the vagus nerve and its impulses to the organs of speech production. Over-action of the vestibular alerts earlier aberrant reflexes. The withdrawal reflexes come into play, and the child cannot talk. The fear paralysis reflex impedes breathing, and affects the muscles for speech, which fall in to a temporary paralysis. The child has the ability to talk— but not in this particular environment. His filtering system for outside stimuli is inadequate. His ability to categorize and discriminate and thus to make sense of his environment is impaired. With this information in mind, the 17 year old girl's descriptions of fear and of breathlessness quoted at the beginning of the paper, start to make sense.

The situation may be further complicated by the presence of one other reflex—the asymmetrical tonic neck reflex (ATNR). Where this persists beyond the normal age of inhibition (6 months of neonate life while awake), several areas of functioning may be impaired. In its primitive form the reflex is elicited as the baby turns its head to one side. The limbs on the side to which the head has turned will extend as the occipital limbs flex. When a child starts to learn fine motor activities such as writing, control of the writing hand will be affected each time that the child turns its head to focus on the writing hand. Hand-eye coordination generally may be immature. Balance may be "thrown" when in the upright position, as any movement of the head in a lateral direction will result in stiffening of the limbs to one side. Smooth eye movements may be affected to the extent that eyes, head and body cannot move independently of one another but can only operate as a unit, so that saccades can only be accomplished with head and/or body tracking. The continued presence of the ATNR will also interfere with the establishment of unilaterality of brain functioning. (Gesell & Ames, 1947) Any task that involves crossing the midline may present difficulties. (Bobath, 1975) A dominant ear and a dominant language center may never have been fully established, so that the child switches erratically from left to right hemisphere for receptive and expressive language tasks.

Both the left and the right hemispheres in the brain have language centers, but the left side is the most efficient for the majority of the population. The left side of the brain is also responsible for the execution of methodical, sequential tasks, while the right side of the brain is responsible for scanning and targeting. If a child has an inadequate filtering mechanism, then the cortex is bombarded by an overload of information which should have been screened earlier in the receiving line. It should have reached the cortex partly categorized, with miscellaneous information filtered out. If this has not occurred, then the left side of the brain will be greatly overworked performing tasks which should have been completed earlier in the receptive process. The processing may then need to switch to the right-brain language center, which the child cannot utilize as immediately or as fluently. The brain may continue switching from righ to left functions. Receiving, processing and the expression of language are not automatic tasks for him in any situation which involves too many stimuli. This child reaches overload far too quickly. With overload comes confusion: confusion generates fear, so that the FPR (fear paralysis reflex) may be activated, and once again the child is unable to speak.

If we return to the earlier DSM III definition of elective mutism, the interpretation may be rather different in the light of these reflexes: "Refusal to speak" may be seen as "inability to speak" and "including at school" may be replaced by "specially at school," where the child does not perceive the environment to be a safe one, because he cannot make sense of it. On the other hand, his willingness to communicate via gestures and nodding starts to seem perfectly reasonable. The associated features also warrant further examination. FPR would induce excessive shyness, social isolation and withdrawal, together with a fear of school. Compulsive traits and negativism tend to be an attempt to establish order and security in an insecure and frightening world. Albeit these are self-defeating strategies for the individual in that situation, they provide some temporary reassurance of self-control in a world that has no safe framework for them in which they could operate effectively. Both DSM III's and DSM IV's apparently incongruous listing of "temper tantrums" as another symptom, presents possibly further manifestation—the second half of the puzzle: a sensory overload comes far too fast for this kind of child.

146

Fear paralysis reflex invokes a state of withdrawal and temporary paralysis. The Moro reflex, on the other hand, elicits an over-reactive response to certain stimuli. Where the fear paralysis reflex remains active in the system at the subcortical level, the Moro reflex will also remain active. (If it does not, then there is no "safety mechanism" to "arouse" the individual from the fear paralysis reflex and in extreme cases, death will result. Sudden infant death syndrome (SIDS) may be one example of this.) Children who have disappeared into the withdrawal state, may only emerge from that state either with a violent outburst of anger, tears of frustration or with hyperactivity. If, finally, the Moro reflex is activated it "releases" them from their paralyzed state. These children are the product of an unresolved conflict between two opposing reflexes, which should not even be present beyond the age of 4 months of neonate life.

Other forms of elective mutism may also be part of this conflict. The individual is unable to verbalize feelings, or to recount events which have a traumatic content. The associated feelings or sensations are so great that the individual becomes imprisoned in a silence which both locks in the feeling and forms part of the pathway to shock. One 11 year old girl later asked: "Why couldn't you see that the way I was, was telling you what I was saying?" as if the silence spoke more loudly and more eloquently than any words could have. In such situations, it is as if the "fight or flight" mechanism is activated, but cannot be released. The fear paralysis traps those sensations inside, before the "fight or flight" mechanism can be used and the internal excitation dispersed. Constant repetition of an "emergency" situation without the ability to fight it, or to run away from it, may result in states of extreme withdrawal (helplessness) and depression, as the activated feelings are turned inward but will not go away. Individuals of this type will find most forms of therapy extremely threatening, as the only release mechanism they know is an explosive and cataclysmic one which they constantly fight to control.

Blythe (1971, 1976) found that the true emotional regressive phase of the hypnotic state would be interrupted if speech was introduced, and the subject was expected to talk during regression. It was as if in the process of speech, the patient lost contact with the feelings. Elective mutism would appear to be the opposite side of the same coin, i.e. where bodily and perceptual sensation is too great, the pathway to speech becomes strangled.

The Institute for Neuro-Physiological Psychology has achieved improvement with a small number of elective mutes on a reflex inhibition program. Initially, the aim has been to stimulate an existing Moro reflex until it is present in its fully retained form. This gives the child a second chance to utilize the Moro reflex—both as an inhibitor to its predecessor, the fear paralysis reflex (FPR) and to give the child the full release mechanisms that it may never have had at any previous stage in its life. Paradoxically, as the Moro reflex reaches its fully retained form, many of the symptoms of overreactivity and oversensitivity actually abate, as if, at last, the body can utilize its instinctive channels of response to danger, to the full.

Brunnström (1962, 1970) may provide one explanation for this. She worked as a physical therapist promoting mobility in children and adults with severe cerebral palsy. She provoked primitive movement patterns which she had observed to be present following either pyramidal tract damage or which are present normally in the fetus. She stated that: *"A patient may be able to perform voluntary flexor and extensor movements, only by utilizing the facilitating effect of one or the other of these reflexes. When a conflict between will and inhibitory reflex impulse exists, the will does not always gain supremacy."*

Finally, the majority of these children have marked vestibular problems.

Vestibular stimulation would seem to be an obvious starting point for a rehabilitation or remediation program. However, as was observed when doing the program as designed at the Institute for Neuro-Physiological Psychology, occupational therapists using the A. Jean Ayres' sensory motor training program, have found that a number of the children who require vestibular stimulation either cannot tolerate it, or only benefit from it to a limited degree. Where the fear paralysis reflex and Moro reflexes are still present, vestibular stimulation may activate one or both of these, so that the patient either finds it too distressing or it reinforces faulty existing compensatory strategies. There may be improvement in gross muscle coordination and balance, but there is rarely a spillover into educational performance. If, however, vestibular stimulation is added <u>after</u> the FPR and Moro reflex have undergone inhibition, the individual is less sensitive, and the program is far more effective, and there will be concomitant improvement in educational performance.

All of the above suggests that there is a physical basis for elective mutism. While accepting that there are cases of both elective mutism and traumatic mutism which are the result of psychological factors, it is nevertheless maintained that for the majority, the psychological factors are of a secondary nature. Where both a fear paralysis reflex (FPR) and a Moro reflex remain active in the individual, certain social situations will present extreme threat. Extreme threat will engender vulnerability in the susceptible individual. Such vulnerability will be accompanied by fear —fear may activate early primitive reflexes at any time in the case of "elective mutism"—paralyzing the organs of speech in specific situations.

DEVELOPMENTAL MILESTONES:
A BLUEPRINT FOR SURVIVAL

SALLY GODDARD N.D.T.

Presented to the Institute for Neuro-Physiological Psychology, November, 1990.

The milestones of life may have been set for us long before we make our entry into the world, but each one should herald our safe arrival from the previous stage of our life, so that we build each stage, block upon solid block. Not everyone is fortunate enough to achieve each milestone. A small percentage will not survive pregnancy. Another percentage will find the process of birth too arduous a journey, and will die during the birth process or shortly afterwards. Another percentage will survive birth and the first hazardous days of life, but may already have had to struggle from conception through pregnancy and birth. They arrive in the world "normal" to all appearances, but with weaknesses in the system which make them vulnerable to a host of minor stressors. It is for this group that each milestone of life may present a threat, or, as Blythe in a 1987 lecture has suggested, it may highlight the basic faults in the system which leave the individual prone to a range of conditions, from sudden infant death syndrome (SIDS) to an inability to cope with stress in later life.

It is upon this specific group that this paper will focus, as it is maintained that their symptoms stem directly from an immaturity in the central nervous system (CNS)and the associated nerve tracts, and its interaction with other systems in the body. Substantiation of this statement will involve the more detailed examination of three systems:

The Reflex System
The Vestibular Apparatus
The Reticular Formation

Every child born into the world should be born with a set of reflexes which are for the infant's survival, and which form the basic reflex system. They start to emerge in utero and should be inhibited, or in certain cases transformed, by a higher part of the brain during pregnancy and the first year of neonate life. If this fails to occur, then they remain aberrant, and they represent a structural weakness in the central nervous system (CNS). The emergence and inhibition of reflexes at the correct time plays a vital role in myelination of the nerves, and it is upon this, that the resulting human being will eventually depend for its efficient functioning at all levels of consciousness.

From the moment of conception the "neural clock" starts to tick, and should continue to do so throughout life. For some people, the clock slips out of kilter very early in development. Though they appear to "make up" the loss and progress through life normally, their ability to function easily and fluently in specific areas may be impaired. The brain and body do not always work in perfect unison. The dysfunction may be barely detectable so that strategies can be used to overcome the problem, but as the stressors become greater, so the compensatory mechanisms start to break down, and the weakness manifests itself. It may appear first in the nursery, the classroom, the playground, or the sportsfield. Often it does not appear until much later, when the adult becomes involved in the more complex processes of life such as career, childbirth, stress and the general demands of modern living. As growing up continues, so more and more systems become involved in a mismatched system of communication. For example: The central nervous system (CNS) may direct incorrect messages to the hypothalamus and the pituitary system, which in turn then—wrongly—influence hormone activity, hunger and satiety, temperature control, libido, and emotions, to name but a few. The reflex structure provides the incorrect blueprint for a complex network of wiring and contacts from one system in the body to another.

The etiology of this syndrome which The Institute for Neuro-Physiological Psychology (INPP) in Chester has termed neuro-developmental delay, is diverse and frequently indeterminate, but it has been suggested that the symptoms which range from clumsiness and ambidexterity, to learning difficulties and emotional disorder, may be hereditary in origin in 50% of the cases, extending back as far as four generations. Eustis (1947) suggested that it is "...characterized by a slow rate of neuromuscular maturation, implying retarded myelination of the motor and associated nerve tracts." Subsequent events may then take their toll, as antenatal problems, difficult birth and injury or illness during the first year of life may instigate or reinforce a preexisting weakness of the central nervous system(CNS). Each system interacting with it then misfires with varying degrees of deviation.

Let us examine how the reflex system provides such a base: The process of normal development is dependent upon the emergence, inhibition and in certain instances, transformation of these primitive reflexes, so that postural reflexes may be released preparing a child for progressive development. "The nervous system learns by doing."(Gilfoyle, Grady & Moore, 1972) and reflexive action aids the continued opening up of neural pathways. Motor behavior should be the product of a system in which brain and body work together to form a communicating system of response, action and expression. Messages should be transmitted with equal efficiency from brain to body and back again, via the efferent and afferent systems. If this is disrupted in any way, then subsequent motor and sensory functions may be affected, altering the transmission of messages from one system in the body to another, and further distorting perceptions, and their transposition from sensory experience into thought, language, emotion, and even the ability to deal with that sensory experience itself. *(See diagram on page 29, Chapter 2)*

It is as if the processing or filtering system in the brain cannot cope with a plethora of information, and therefore "cuts out" at a very crude level. It is bombarded by conflicting sensory stimuli which it cannot categorize immediately, and it becomes overloaded far too quickly.

The first area of sensory response to develop in utero is the tactile response, and its realization may be observed in the primitive withdrawal reflex which first appears between 5 and 7 weeks after conception. Early avoidance reflexes —and Gilfoyle, Grady & Moore state that there are many of them in the first few weeks of uterine life— form the basis of the developing reflex structure. Capute (1986) says that these very early reflexes emerge in utero and should be inhibited in utero: that they should have been controlled by higher centers in the fetal development system before later reflexes in utero can develop fully.

At 9 weeks after conception, as the withdrawal reflexes are being controlled, the Moro reflex should start to emerge. Both the vestibular system and the cerebellum are also developing at this time. Let us suppose, that at this dynamic stage in development, either as a result of faulty genetic programming, or some current uterine or external anomaly, something shifts imperceptibly out of phase. The avoidance reflexes remain active in the chain instead of being inhibited by the developing Moro reflex at 9-12 weeks gestation. The Moro reflex itself then fails to develop fully. Subsequent reflexes emerge, and fulfill their function to a degree, but they remain "locked" in the system, neither fully aiding the embryo through each stage in development, nor undergoing full inhibition at the appropriate time.

Because they may not persist in a retained form, they remain undetected, and the resulting person is deemed medically to be "normal." There is a basic weakness in the system, however, which will exact a price later at the conscious level, for the tasks which should be automatic, have not become so.

The reflex system is built in a sequence with each reflex playing both a facilitatory and an inhibitory role in the reflex chain. The Landau reflex, for example, aids inhibition of the tonic labyrinthine reflex (TLR), and Capute has suggested that the symmetrical tonic neck reflex (STNR) may be a part of the process of the tonic labyrinthine (TLR) undergoing transformation. Thus, a correct sequence from the beginning is a vital precursor to the development of the central nervous system, as well as motor, perceptual, cognitive and emotional development. Each reflex affects a specific area of functioning. Different combinations of aberrant reflexes will build different pictures, different problems and different people.

The question that poses itself here is: How can three of the earliest reflexes impair later functioning and affect other systems in the body if they remain "locked" in the chain?

The withdrawal reflex which, first appears at 5-7 weeks after conception, is initially a rapid amebic-like withdrawal movement of the whole organism as a response to touch in the oral region. A few days later the head will turn away from the stimulus, and by the end of the 12th week the eyes will close—tightly shut—as an additional response.

It has been suggested (Goddard, 1989), that these early withdrawal reflexes may be the earliest manifestation of a fear paralysis reflex (FPR), described in detail by Kaada (1986), as a major factor in sudden infant death syndrome (SIDS). He describes many of its characteristics in infancy, where it may be recognized as the "terrified rabbit," who becomes frozen to the spot at which he has first experienced sudden fear. Kaada describes its features, beginning with an immediate motor paralysis accompanied by respiratory arrest in expiration, reduced muscle tone, lack of response to external stimuli, activation of a pain-suppressing mechanism and bradycardia with peripheral vasoconstriction. It may be accompanied by an increase in systolic pressure and pulse pressure combined with muscle hypotonia. It represents a maladaptive response to situations with which the individual is unable to cope.

The Moro reflex has been described as the "first primitive shock response." (Bennett, 1988) It should be inhibited by three months of neonate life, and then transformed into the adult startle reflex or Strauss reflex. It has also been described as the initiator of the "fight or flight" mechanism as its activation stimulates the sympathetic nervous system in preparation for what it interprets to be a life threatening event. The Moro reflex demands instant reflexive response, irrespective of the source of real or imagined danger. Bennett suggested that its continued presence beyond three months of neonate life, is a major factor in anxiety states, as the individual remains hypersensitive to minor stimuli and the Moro demands an overreactive response. Here, the limbic system switches to "emergency" before the cortex has time to filter out the source of distress and to direct a rational response.

In the neonate, the Moro reflex appears as a violent, distressed reflex. Arms and legs will convulsively extend, freeze fractionally, and then adduct. As the limbs go out, the head will be thrown back and there will be a massive intake of breath in preparation for the lifesaving scream.

If this reflex persists beyond three to four months of neonate life, it will result in a degree of hypersensitivity and over reactivity, depending upon its strength. If it is only residually present in those first few months of life, the implications may be rather different. The reflex may be weak in its entirety, or, the second part of the reflex may be underdeveloped or even absent. In that case, although there may be a massive intake of breath, the ensuing adduction of the arms and the releasing of the breath cannot take place. This would result in respiratory arrest in expiration so that breathing appears to "freeze" and the baby's cry for help is never uttered. The baby becomes captured in the "freeze" state —the possible remnant of the fear paralysis reflex (FPR). It is not dissimilar to the experience of "dry drowning," which can occur if someone is thrown unexpectedly into extremely cold water. Everything in the body "locks" from the shock of the cold, so that it is impossible to expand or contract the lungs —either to inhale or to exhale breath. Within a very short time it is possible to drown in this way, without any water ever entering the lungs.

Cottrell (1987) became interested in a correlation between asthma and the continued presence of the Moro reflex. He stated: "All primitive reflexes require a compensation mechanism from higher centers of the brain. The Moro, being a startle reflex, requires an overriding effect. The adult version of the "fight or flight" response is more sophisticated and will, whenever possible, be given priority by the body. This requires several differing types of compensations. First, is the necessity to restore the normal mechanism of controlling the muscular reaction. Second, is the need to produce adrenaline reaction to any frightening situation. This is done through lowering the stimulus threshold, which makes for a very frightened individual who is hypersensitive and overresponds to every threat."

"Where there is a retained or residual Moro, the CO_2 reflex does not develop. The combination between that lack of CO_2 and the need to keep the individual from taking that deep breath, leads to shallow apical breathing, and frequently to hyperventilation —an important precursor to panic."

Cottrell's observations touch on three important areas: respiratory functioning, rigid control of muscle tone and adrenal output. Each one of these may play a vital instigating and/or a sustaining role in panic disorders and a range of other conditions for which there appears to be no adequate pathology, and which are therefore regarded as "psychosomatic illnesses." Gold (1986) described one aspect of this: "When the child's cortex gets into overload, it sends messages to the adrenal gland and the pituitary. All they can tell is that they got a signal to squirt out their chemicals. Each time, when they get the signal the adrenals squirt out adrenaline and cortisol. Pretty soon the adrenals get exhausted. As the adrenals get exhausted, allergies start to show up along with psychosomatic illnesses, headaches, migraines, colitis ulcers and high blood pressure. Hay Fever is one of the symptoms."

Odent (1984) describes part of this syndrome another way. He outlines Laborit's (1952) concept of "inhibition of action," a term used to describe a basically submissive behavioral pattern. This is a direct result of an inability to respond to a stressful situation by either fight or flight. In experiments on rats, Laborit was able to trace the origin of high blood pressure to just such situations of continuous frustration.

Odent's hormonal studies confirm Laborit's theory: "Inhibition of action generates the secretion of noradrenaline and cortisol; cortisol itself triggers the inhibition of action the result being a vicious circle ... noradrenaline contracts the blood vessels, quickens the heartbeat, and raises the blood pressure, and cortisol has many kinds of long term effects, such as depressing the immune system and destroying the thymus."

Odent links continuous hormonal reactions to pathogenic situations of this kind, as major factors in the etiology of psychosomatic diseases. It is therefore of interest that both the withdrawal reflexes and the Moro reflex exert a direct influence upon these reaction patterns.

The third reflex I would like to look at, which takes a leading role in the interplay between the systems in the body, is the tonic labyrinthine reflex (TLR). It is thought that this reflex also emerges in recognizable form towards the end of the first trimester of pregnancy. Capute (1986) suggests that flexus habitus itself may be a manifestation of the TLR forwards, but the TLR backwards may not be fully activated for the first time until the baby's head goes into extension before entering the birth canal. (Machover, 1990) This may be one reason why the full reflex in both flexion and extension is generally not accepted to be present until after birth. The tonic labyrinthine reflex (TLR) is the infant's only way of reacting to gravity, and is normally present in its crude form by 3 months of neonate life. If the baby is lying on its back with the trunk supported, then the reflex may be elicited by allowing the head to drop back below the midline. This will result in an extensor thrust of the arms and the legs. If the head is then brought forward above the midline, the baby will start to curl up into a fetal position. If the reflex is still active when the baby makes the transition to toddler, then the head righting reflexes, which are essential to sit and to stand, will be impaired and the balance will be affected when in the upright position. Any movement of the head too far forwards or backwards will result in either reflexive flexion or reflexive extension of the limbs. Only through conscious muscular effort and in direct conflict with the reflexive response, can these movements be controlled.

What happens if we try to act in direct opposition to a normal reflexive response? Imagine that you have touched a scalding kettle. The immediate natural reaction is to withdraw the hand as quickly as possible. If you deliberately act against this reflex, what happens? The obvious result is that the hand gets burned, but what are the other reactions in the body? There is a change in breathing, increase in heart rate, and tightening of all the muscles in the body as the body "armors" itself against the natural reaction. When at last you do "give way" to the reflex there is relief, a feeling of fatigue and probably little knowledge of what else has occurred in the immediate environment during the period of time that you have been fighting the reflex. Individuals with a cluster of aberrant reflexes have to perform this ritual in every moment of their waking lives in order to function normally. In extreme, there is a choice of only two directions to cope: either hyperactivity, as a means of keeping the system "on the go," or withdrawal. This choice may have to be made in one or several areas of life to avoid the most difficult or sensitive situations.

The tonic labyrinthine reflex also exerts a direct influence upon the labyrinth. The labyrinth is a complex organ for attaining balance, which, by movement of fluid in three orthogonal tubes operates rather like a spirit level, activating special nerves which send signals to the brain concerning movement of the head. The vestibular apparatus then detects changes of direction and position of the head in space, particularly when the movement starts and stops. It also records the amount of forwards, backwards or sideways tilting of the head, as well as its movement when the whole body moves in a linear direction. Odent suggests that it is the vestibular organ which directs the fetus' orientation in utero, and deficiencies in its function might result in breech or shoulder presentations at birth. Information from the vestibular apparatus is combined with information from other sensory channels. Both pre-natally and post-natally the vestibular system controls body image impression and reinforcement, and also kinesthesia—the sensation of bodily movement in space. If a strong tonic labyrinthine reflex (TLR) persists, then balance will be constantly "thrown." Messages received by the vestibular will be inaccurate and fluctuating. The cortex will have to perform a detective task in decoding which messages are relevant and which are irrelevant.

One example of the cortex at work can be seen in cases of auditory delay, or auditory confusion. The ear acts as a collecting organ not only for sound stimuli, but also for those stimuli that are responsible for coordinating the vestibular portion of the labyrinth. (Tomatis 1980) If the vestibular, as a result of aberrant reflexes, is receiving conflicting messages from other sensory channels, its processing may be impaired. The confusion may make it unable to relay sound messages received from the ear to the language processing centers in the cortex. Another example may be seen in some autistic children who fail to respond to communication through the auditory channel, although there is no evidence of hearing loss. These children may already be in such a state of internal excitation and arousal that, to cope at all, they have to amputate one system from their consciousness.

Activation of the tonic labyrinthine reflex (TLR) involves both the vestibular apparatus and the reticular formation. The reticular formation is net-like in appearance and is situated in the central part of the brain stem. It operates as the basis of an alerting system, by sending messages to the cerebral cortex and the afferent pathways, in order to maintain the brain in a condition in which consciousness can occur. The ascending pathways have an arousing function, while the descending pathways—via the reticulospinal tract—influence the neuron pools. The facilitatory area fires spontaneously, but the inhibitory area (which has a sedating affect), relies on the basal ganglia, cerebellum and cortex. It is stated in Merck (1987) that: "the alert state requires an instant interaction between the cognitive functions of the cerebral hemispheres and the arousal mechanisms of the reticular formation."

If the reticular formation fails to act appropriately, then unconsciousness can be the result. Within the reticular formation are areas which regulate the cardiovascular, respiratory, endocrine and gastrointestinal systems. Emotions also come under its influence through the limbic system and hypothalamus. Brain (1987), suggests that epilepsy may be one result of a misfiring in the reticular formation, the origins stemming back to an immaturity within the central nervous system (CNS), which lowers the threshold to seizure.

In the light of this, it may be possible to devise a schema, whereby a misfiring in the brainstem as a direct result of aberrant reflexes results in either extreme over-excitation (hyperactivity), or under-stimulation (the cutting out of one or more sensory channels until eventual total unconsciousness is the outcome) i.e. the filtering mechanism is not doing its job. Instead of sifting and dumping irrelevant information and stimuli, it allows everything to pass through to higher centers in the brain. This would either heighten arousal to an abnormal level, or it would close the gate entirely, so that the system goes into "shut down."

In what circumstances might this "shut down" operate? Epilepsy may be one, where the threshold to seizure is low as a result of immaturity within the central nervous system. Fay (1942) even went so far as to describe an epileptic fit as, "a defense reflex" which attempts by convulsive efforts to regain a favorable formula or a state of equilibrium. There are, of course, varying types and degrees of seizure, not all of which can be categorized as "epileptic." At this point I would like to look further at how "seizure-like" episodes may stem from withdrawal reflexes remaining active in the nervous system chain. The result would be an inadequate interaction between the vestibular apparatus, reticular activating system and cerebellum, with subsequent impairment to the arousal mechanisms.

Southall, Samuels & Talbert (1990), have recently produced a study on the incidence of cyanotic episodes in potential sudden infant death syndrome (SIDS) babies and those who actually became SIDS victims. Many of the symptoms they describe bear a remarkable resemblance to the features of the fear paralysis reflex (Kaada, 1986) and to the "seizure-like" episodes experienced by adults for which no adequate medical explanation can be found. Tests may have been carried out for a number of conditions such as diabetes, hypoglycemia, epilepsy, thyroid malfunction and even for tumors, with none of these being detected. Southall, Samuels & Talbert (1990) describe cyanotic episodes which occur at a median age of 7 weeks of neonate life, when the Moro reflex should be at its height. They note that the most common trigger was a sudden naturally occurring stimulus from pain, fear or anger, most often in the form of a sudden shock. In their studies they found no evidence of actual seizure activity, but episodes were more common when the infant was tired (reduced ability to compensate for the weakness), when there was a high level of emotional tension in the home, or when the routine of the infant was interrupted. Infection, particularly respiratory infection, increased the frequency and severity of the episodes.

These episodes commonly began with a series of attempts at expiratory cries without inspiratory effort and with a widely open mouth. If crying became established, the attack was unlikely to develop further. If it did not, then within 30 seconds unconsciousness would ensue accompanied either by opisthotonus or tonic convulsion, or both. At the beginning of the episode the heart rate would rise to above 170 beats per minute (B.P.M.) dropping dramatically to around 80 B.P.M. as bradycardia progressed. Now, let us examine how these symptoms may link with Kaada's description of the fear paralysis reflex (FPR) outlined earlier. Kaada describes it as "a reflex present in the entire animal kingdom, which is temporarily released from cortical control as a result of extreme fear." It is accompanied by bradycardia which acts as disinhibitory phenomenon and is the final manifestation of a common pathway to shock. The reflex when activated leaves no trace of itself in the organism, so that no adequate cause can be established for the cessation of breathing and pulmonary effort. If the fear paralysis reflex remains active at the subcortical level, then the Moro reflex cannot operate fully to open the airways, or to allow exhalation in moments of extreme crisis. If this is added to a heightened sensibility to shock, the results may be fatal. Southall, Samuels & Talbert suggest a definite link between brain-stem defects, including disturbances to the respiratory generators, to the centers controlling pulmonary vasomotor tone, and to the processing of reflexes arising in the pulmonary vascular bed or lung. Thus, a misfiring in the brainstem from those reflexes which influence breathing, circulation and arousal may be responsible for a number of behaviors. Lack of adequate arousal may be a result, not of under sensitivity, but of hypersensitivity, where the threshold of tolerance to external stimuli is abnormally low. In such cases, even touching may be painful and many bodily sensations a torment rather than a reassurance or a pleasure.

Certain autistic behaviors can be linked to sensory input overload of this kind. Many autistic children cannot tolerate wearing clothes, and most of them will remove their shoes and socks whenever possible. Many are excessively ticklish and cannot stand even simple daily routines such as being dried with a towel. Eating may present problems, as they detest either very smooth or very chewy food and may insist on a narrow, repetitive diet. It has been observed (O'Reilly, 1989) that they appear to be more responsive after vigorous exercise, and some of their autistic symptoms lessen during episodes of diarrhea and vomiting, prolonged fasting, or —if they are epileptic— after an epileptic episode. It is as if they attempt to raise, artificially, the arousal mechanisms which they need to function, and to maintain their performance at a more alert level. Both exercise and fasting have long been recognized as producing mild states of euphoria. Vomiting and diarrhea alter the body chemistry, leaving a heightened concentration of insulin active in the system, as the body normally produces insulin in response to any intake of food. Under normal conditions, food is consumed and converted into glucose which is utilized by the body for energy, and gradually the blood glucose level drops. Where excessive exercise has taken place, or bouts of vomiting or diarrhea have occurred, there will be too great a concentration of insulin left in the blood, as the blood glucose level will drop much faster. Lowering of the blood glucose level stimulates the secretions of the adrenal glands whose hormones have the opposite effect to insulin. These hormones are passed in the blood to the liver, where they facilitate the conversion of stored glycogen into glucose, balancing the action of insulin so that in normal health an optimum blood sugar level is maintained. Adrenaline secreted by the adrenal center should produce a similar "balancing" effect, but its rate of use is rather different. It forms part of the emergency system which stimulates a rapid glucose increase to provide a sudden energy surge, but which also plunges the individual into a state of hyper-awareness and hyper-responsiveness a state of artificially induced hormonal arousal. Certain cases of anorexia and bulimia may also be part of this vicious cycle. Stress alone can cause dramatic fluctuations in blood sugar level as emotional aggravation induces a rise in blood sugar to deal with the immediate crisis. The rise in blood sugar is then countered by increased insulin secretion with a subsequent fall in blood sugar—another vicious cycle is set in motion.

At its most extreme, the continued presence of the withdrawal reflexes may result in death or unconsciousness, but other permutations are also possible. The withdrawal reflexes may remain active in the chain at the suppressed level. The Moro reflex develops and functions normally for a percentage of the time, but does not always have an over-riding effect over the withdrawal reflexes. Both remain active in the system beyond the normal age of inhibition, performing a juggling feat as to which exerts priority. In certain instances both reflexes will be overcome by conscious control, and the individual will respond to a situation rationally and effectively. At other times (frequently when the individual is tired), the situation may provoke the Moro reflex, and an over-reaction response. On another occasion the withdrawal reflexes will claim priority, and the individual my find it impossible to respond at all. One example of this interplay between control and the reflexes may be seen in cases of so-called elective mutism. A child may be loquacious and articulate in one environment (usually the home environment), but when placed in a less familiar or less secure setting will refuse to respond verbally to any form of communication. Both the terms "elective mutism" and "refuse to respond" infer that the child chooses to remain silent on these occasions. What is far more probable, is that the child cannot speak in these settings.

Let us take a hypothetical case and examine how a reflex profile might impair the mechanisms of speech under certain conditions: A child reaches the age of 7 with a reflex profile as follows: a residually present Moro reflex, a residually present asymmetrical tonic neck reflex and a virtually retained tonic labyrinthine reflex. He is hypersensitive to sound and to touch. His balance is unstable, his headrighting reflexes are under-developed, and thus his spatial awareness and orientation skills are poor. He is stimulus bound, and his eyes do not always work as they should.

Each day, when he goes to school, he walks into an environment which, at best, is buzzing with noise, movement and activity. At its worst, it is a conglomerate of individual sounds which ebb and flow from continuous background noise. He cannot discriminate, categorize and occlude miscellaneous noise or movement immediately, because he does not have an automatic filtering mechanism for the auditory, visual or proprioceptive channels. He has either to attend to outside stimuli or to dismiss them through a conscious and methodical route. Both the left and the right hemispheres, in the brain, have language centers, but the most efficient is on the left side for the majority of the population. It is the left side of the brain which is responsible for the execution of methodical, sequential tasks, while the right side of the brain is responsible for scanning and targeting. For example, if you were seeking out a face in a crowd, the left brain would go through every face in the crowd in order, until it found the one it was looking for. The right brain would scan the faces until it hit on its target. For children without an adequate filtering mechanism, the left brain is being greatly overworked, and they may need to switch to the right brain (subdominant) language center which they cannot utilize as fluently. The environment of noise and strange place is, therefore, a very frightening one for this child.

The vestibular apparatus is constantly monitoring, adjusting and correcting. It is also linked to the l0th or vagus nerve at the level of the medulla (Blythe, 1990). This vagus nerve contains two sets of fibers.

1. Sensory fibers which carry messages to part of the external ear, and afferent messages from the pharynx, larynx and thoracic and abdominal viscera.

2. Motor fibers and accessory nerves, which serve the striated muscles of the palate, larynx and pharynx.

This child is already overloaded by stimuli, and his compensatory mechanisms are stretched to capacity. Too much energy is taken up in attempting to regulate incoming stimuli, and he has little left for expression. The overworked vestibular excites the vagus nerve and its impulses to the organs of speech production. Overreaction of the vestibular also alerts earlier aberrant reflexes. Now the withdrawal reflexes come into play, and he cannot talk. In order to function at all in other areas, speech is eliminated entirely, until either he reaches an environment in which he can relax his controls, or, until the level of overload becomes so great that the Moro is activated, releasing an explosive expressive reaction.

A similar reaction pattern may be seen in cases of emotional stress where the individual is unable to verbalize feelings or to recount events which have a traumatic content. The associated feelings are so great, that the individual becomes imprisoned in a state of emotional mutism or hysterical paralysis, as part of the pathway to shock. The words of expression may be frantically circulating inside the head, but the feelings are so overwhelming that the person cannot release the mechanisms to speech. One 11 year old girl asked later, when her problems had been resolved, "Why couldn't you see that the way I was, was telling you what I was saying?" A burst of anger, or a flood of tears may open the gateway to speech, as the Moro is finally activated to release from the partly paralyzed state.

Hypersensitivity with a lowered threshold to shock was suggested as one pathway. The overloaded system goes into "shutdown" in one or more sensory channels in order to cope. The other pathway outlined was that resulting from a lowered arousal threshold, which catapults the system into an increasing state of arousal and over-activity.

Where there is arousal, internal excitation and muscle tension increase. Where there is prolonged muscle tension, eventually there is fatigue. Fatigue will reduce performance, so that in order to maintain the same level of performance and make up the loss of efficiency, there will need to be an increased level of arousal. Thus, a vicious circle is created, in which over-activity of body musculature becomes both a survival and a performance system. Tiredness becomes an enemy to be overcome, not by rest and restoration, but by increased movement and activity like changing gear up, as the revs increase. A crisis is reached when after topgear and overdrive, there are no further gears to change up to, but somehow the same level of performance has to be maintained. This may be achieved temporarily by boosting adrenaline in the system, whether it be through drugs, more excitement, or by violent outbursts in the form of anger, extreme depression or states of elation. These individuals may be hypersensitive to drugs and to alcohol, to the extent that the drugs actually have the opposite effect to the normal one.

It has been recognized for a number of years that certain hyperactive children react badly to mild sedatives such as Phenergan (Avomine) and Vallergan. Far from calming them down, these drugs will throw them into a state of heightened aggression and distress. These children need their constant activity to keep them going. Momentum and movement are means of survival— by sedating these, you take away the only way they know of functioning. If given a stimulant such as Ritalin (Dextroamphetamine) you actually help them to perform to their level —without the constant need for self-induced overarousal.

It has been found in a number of cases by the Institute for Neuro-Physiological Psychology that, if you increase the Moro until it is present for a short time in its fully retained form, many of the symptoms of fatigue and over-excitation actually diminish. It is as if, by allowing the subject to use the primitive "fight or flight" mechanism to its fullest, the internal tension and excitation is released, until the primitive Moro reflex is no longer required by the body and, together with other reflex abnormalities, the Moro can undergo transformation. As greater automatic control is achieved within the body, so many of the presenting symptoms remiss.

To summarize: Analysis of the reflex system provides signposts to the functioning of the central nervous system (CNS) as the reflexes provide the foundation for a mature CNS, which then interlinks with all other systems in the body.

It is here suggested that early damage to the Reflex Sequence may lead to dysfunctions in the Vestibular Apparatus and the Reticular Formation, resulting in either <u>over-sedation</u> (as in Sudden Infant Death Syndrome, Epilepsy, seizure-like episodes, and certain autistic behaviors) or at the other extreme, <u>over-arousal</u>, where certain panic disorders or "neurotic" states may be the outcome.

WHY DO OUR CHILDREN ROLL AND TUMBLE?

By Sally Goddard

Published in "First Steps" magazine, Australia.

The first of all the senses to develop, is the sense of balance. It is vital for posture, movement, and a sense of "center" in space, time, motion, depth and self. All other sensation passes through the balance mechanism (vestibular system) at brainstem level before it is passed on to its specialized region higher in the brain. Hence, all the other senses which a child will depend upon for learning are linked to balance.

To the newborn baby, perception and motion are the same thing. He is not aware that sound and movement, vision and touch are separate sensations, as for him they all fuse together as a single experience or feeling. Thus motion is the child's first language, and the more eloquent he becomes in his primary language, the quicker he will develop other powers of expression, exploration and development.

Stimulation of the balance mechanism is an integral part of the embryo's growth from the moment of conception. Every movement that the mother makes is felt in the cushioned environment of the womb. After birth the feelings continue to be sensed through a vast repertoire of movement patterns from lying, kicking, rolling and sitting, to crawling and creeping on the hands and knees, walking, running hopping, skipping, swinging, rolling and tumbling. It is through movement that further connections are made between the vestibular apparatus and higher centers of the brain. It takes until the age of 7 - 8 years for the balance mechanism, the cerebellum and the corpus callosum to be myelinated, and it is during these early years that vestibular stimulation is the natural ingredient in every normal child's play.

The infant begins with constant repetition of arm and leg movements, practicing extension and flexion of the muscles and training hand-eye coordination. The eight-month-old who rolls back and forth across the floor with no particular goal in sight, is preparing her balance for sitting, standing and eventually walking. As far as she is concerned, when she moves, the world moves with her, and when she stops the world stands still once more. Creeping on hands and knees then acts as an important bridge, enabling her to combine the use of her vestibular, proprioceptive and visual systems for the first time. Walking then increases not only mobility, but allows her to roam with independent use of the hands. These are the early building blocks for learning which must then be practiced and integrated with other systems. Thus, in the early years, movement is the child's main vocabulary and language is body based. Voluntary control of movement can only develop though the broadening of movement horizons.

The 3-6 year old child who constantly hops, skips and twirls while "walking" down the street, is still learning to control her balance, for the most advanced level of balance is the ability stay still. The action of NOT moving requires whole body functions and muscle groups to operate together without continuous adjustment, and signifies the advent of mature postural control. The child who cannot stay still, instinctively knows that her balance still needs practice. The child who cannot stay on the sidewalk if there is a low wall running alongside it, but who must climb from one level to another and back again, is still teaching herself muscle control, depth perception and visualmotor integration skills. Somersaults and cartwheels further facilitate the separation of motion from other sensations, for it is only when a child has control of movement that she can pay attention to other experiences.

Hyperactivity and Attention Deficit may be two signs of immaturity in vestibular functioning. As parents, teachers and caretakers, we tend to implore our hyperactive children to "sit still" and to "be quiet." It has been shown that hyperactive children who are allowed to spin for 30 seconds in either direction, show increased attention span for up to 30 minutes afterwards, suggesting that they need vestibular stimulation to "get their brain into gear."

Our eyes operate from the vestibular circuit in the brain. Our ears share the same cranial nerve and the sense of touch is integrally linked to the vestibular through the movement across hair cells whose receptors are located in the dermis of the skin. If motion is a child's first language, then sensation is his second. Only when both motion and sensation are integrated can the higher language skills of speech, reading and writing develop fluently. Our children who roll and tumble are engaged in their first lesson toward becoming the Einsteins of the future.

Other papers and articles by Sally Goddard Blythe: **www.inpp.org.uk**

Appendix 3

Glossary

Accommodation: ability to focus quickly from near to far distance and vice versa.

Afferent: information leading to the brain.

Apraxia: see praxis.

Babkin response: The stimulus for this reflex consists of deep pressure, applied simultaneously to the palms of both hands while the infant is an appropriate position, ideally supine. The stimulus is followed by flexion or forward bowing of the head, opening of the mouth and closing of the eyes. The reflex can be demonstrated in the newborn, but should be inhibited after four months of age. It shows a neurological link between the mouth and the hands, which also becomes obvious in the palming movements of the hands a child makes while nursing. (Kittens do this when being fed.) Like many reflexes, it can be elicited in either direction.

Balance system: monitors all sensation in both directions.

Basal Ganglia: Three small masses of nerve tissue —the caudate nucleus, the putamen and the globus pallidus. Located at the base of the brain, they are involved in the subconscious regulation of movements.

Bradycardia: slow heartbeat rate.

Cephalo-caudal law: from head downward sequel of development in the infant.

Crawling: moving forward using arms and legs with belly and chest on the ground. (Crawling on tummy)

Creeping: crawling on hands and knees.

dB (decibels): measure of volume of sound.

Dermis: Top layer of the skin.

Dominance: Supremacy of one side over another within the brain. This refers to the two cerebral hemispheres, but it can be applied to other parts of the body, where there are two of each. E.g. the hands, ears, eyes, feet, etc.

Dyslexia: Inability to read. Generally used only in cases where there is normal intelligence, but where the usual methods of teaching have failed.

Dyspraxia (or apraxia): the inability to select responses in an appropriate order and orient them for proper execution, even though no paralysis exists.

Extension: Movement away from the body.

Efferent: information or commands from the central nervous system to the body.

Figure ground effect: inability to separate and categorize conflicting visual information, e.g. walking up an open staircase or crossing a slatted bridge, where the water can be seen through the boards.

Flexion: bending toward the front center of the body.

Fixation: focusing of eyes on a stationary point and holding that focus.

Hyper: oversensitive, inadequate filtering of extraneous sensations.

Hypertonus: extensor muscles exert greater influence than the flexor muscles.

Hypo: undersensitive, inadequate sensations received.

Hypotonus: weak muscle tone.

Hz: Hertz vibrations per second, determine the pitch of the sound heard. E.g. 125 Hz is low sound, 8000 Hz is perceived as high sound.

In utero: in the mother's womb.

Kinesthesis: see proprioception.

Lateral line receptor: a sensory system found in many kinds of fish and some amphibians that informs the animal of water motion in relation to body surface.

Limbic system: Part of the old cortex and its primary related nuclei. It is shared by all mammals and is associated with smell, autonomic functions and certain aspects of emotion and behavior.

Midbrain: the uppermost part of the brain stem. The term midbrain is sometimes used to include all the structures just below the cortex, sometimes even including the cerebellum.

Muscle tone: balance between flexion and extension muscles.

Myelin: a soft fatty substance surrounding a nerve fiber.

Neuro-developmental delay: The presence of primitive reflexes beyond their normal age of inhibition and/or the absence of postural reflexes.

Opisthotonus: A form of spasm in which the head and heels are bent backward and the body bowed forward.

Parasympathetic nervous system: increases salivary gland secretions, decreases the heart rate, promotes digestion and dilates the blood vessels. It is the opposite partner of the sympathetic nervous system.

Praxis: the brain's ability to select responses, arrange them in an appropriate order and orient them for proper execution.

Proprioception: ability to know where different parts of the body are and to carry out complex maneuvers without conscious awareness. Though often used interchangeably with kinesthesis, the term proprioception encompasses all sensations involving body position, either at rest or in motion, the term kinesthesia refers only to sensations arising when active muscle contraction becomes involved.

Reflex: involuntary movement in response to a stimulus and the entire physiological process activitating it.

Reflex Inhibition Program: A series of exercises based upon fetal and infant movement patterns. Its purpose is to inhibit aberrant primitive reflexes and is tailored specifically to the needs of each individual.

Reticular Activating System: A complex network of nerve fibers, occupying the central core of the brain stem, that function in wakefullness and alertness.

Simian: ape-like.

Saccades: rapid eye movements which accuratedly take the eye from fixation point to fixation point when a person reads a line of text. Saccadic eye movement also serves the function of erasing the prior visual image.

Scoliosis: abnormal curvature of the spine.

Sympathetic nervous system: network of nerve fibers which, especially under stress, ready the body for either flight or standing to fight. It does so by increasing the heartbeat, quickening the breath and enhancing the supply of oxygen to the muscles by syphoning the blood supply from the skin to deep muscle. It works in a balancing act with the parasympathetic nervous system to keep the body in a state of metabolic equilibrium.

Tactile defensive: touch receptors respond to stimulation as if it were a threat.

Threshold: the point at which a stimulus is strong enough to cross over a synapse.

Ventral: lying or supported on tummy, head and hips not supported.

White noise: continuous background sensation, which is always present and intrudes upon other sensations. Can be an auditory, a visual or a tactile sensation.

Appendix 4

Useful Addresses

The Institute for Neuro-Physiological Psychology is responsible for the research, training*, and clinical practice of methods developed at INPP.

The Institute for Neuro-Physiological Psychology (INPP)
4, Stanley Place
Chester CH1 2LU UK
Email: inpp@virtual-chester.net
Website: www.inpp.org.uk

INPP Scotland
Sheila Dobie
20 High Street
South Queensferry
Edinburgh EH30 4PP

In addition to the main training course for professionals who wish to practice INPP's methods, INPP also runs one-day courses in the use of a small test battery and series of developmental exercises that can be used in schools with small or large groups of children. A number of INPP trained practitioners are licensed to teach this course.

The International School for Research and Training in Neuro-Developmental Delay (ISND) is responsible for the training of all professionals wishing to use the reflex stimulation and inhibition programs devised by The Institute for Neuro-Physiological Psychology. ISND is represented in Sweden, Germany, Ireland and Finland.

For further information on training courses and seminars, contact:

The International School for Research and Training in Neuro-Developmental Delay
4, Stanley Place
Chester CH1 2LU UK
Email: inpp@virtual-chester.net
Website: www.inpp.org.uk

ISND courses outside of the UK:

Sweden
The Swedish Institute for Neuro-Physiological Psychology
Catharina Johannesson Alvegård
Rydholmasgat.42
S41873, Gothenberg. Sweden.

Germany
ISND Deutschland.
Thake Hansen-Lauff
Katzbek 14
24235 Laboe
Germany
Email:Hansen-lauff@inpp.de
Website: www.inpp.DE

Ireland
ISND Ireland
Mary O' Connor
Balrickyard
Galway Road
Headford
Co. Galway.
Ireland
Email: mfoc@eircom.net

Finland
Veli and Nina Laurinsalo
Ylipalontie 7 B 4
00670 Helsinki
Finland

Other Centers practicing INPP's methods:

United States of America

Dr. Lawrence J. Beuret
4811 Emerson, Suite 209
Palatine, Illinois 60067 U.S.A.

Sweden

Sensomotoriskt Centrum
Håkan Carlsson
Blakintskolan
Martensgaten 12
595 32 Mjolby. Sweden

Netherlands
in cooperation with:
Marjolein Aarten-Willemse
Van Ruysdaellaan 37
2264TK Leidschendam
Netherlands

Jur Ten Hoopen
Amsteldyk 138
1079 LE Amsterdam
Netherlands
Website: www.inpp.NL

Germany

Deutsche Gesellschaft neurophysiologischer Entwicklungsförderer e.V.
Katzbek 14
24235 Laboe
Germany

Other Centers Specializing in Child Development:

Australia
ANSUA - Children's Learning & Development Centre
Maureen Hawke
333 Given Terrace
Rosalie
Queensland, Australia   *www.ansua.org.au*

SOUND THERAPY CENTERS

Dyslexia Research Laboratory
Dr. Kjeld Johansen
Rö Skolovej 14 DK 3760
Gudhjem. Bornholm. Denmark
Email: kvj@dyslexic-lab.dk

The Tomatis Centre UK Ltd
3 Wallands Crescent
Lewes
East Sussex BN7 2QT UK

The Listening Centre
Paul Madaule
599 Markham Street
Toronto, Canada M6G 2L7
Email: listen@idirect.com

Auditory Integrative Training (Dr. Guy Berard)
Information available from:
The Georgiana Foundation
PO Box 2607
Westport, CT 06880 USA

Samonas (Dr. I Steinbach)
Klangstudio LAMBDOMA
Markgrafenufer 9
59071 Hamm.Germany

The Listening Programme
Alex Doman, Advanced Brain Technologies
PO Box 1088
Ogden, Utah 84402 USA

OPTOMETRY

For further information
addresses available from:

Optometric Extension Program
Foundation Inc.
Vision West Inc.
1921 E Carnegie Avenue
Suite 3L
Santa Ana, CA 92705 USA

College of Optometrists in Vision
Development
PO Box 285
Chula Vista, CA 91912-0285

READING DIFFICULTIES

The ARROW Trust
Dr. Colin Lane
The Priory Annexe
St Mary's Street
Bridgewater
Somerset TA6 3EK
Website: www.self-voice.co.uk

AUTISM
Autism Research Institute
Bernard Rimland, Ph.D.
4182 Adams Avenue
San Diego, CA 92116 USA

Appendix 5

References

American Psychiatric Association, (1994) Diagnostic and Statistical Manual of Mental Disorders.(DSM IV) Washington, DC.

American Psychiatric Association, (1980) DSM III, Washington DC.

Ames, L. Bates, (1967) Is your child in the wrong grade? Harper and Rowe, New York.

André-Thomas, Saint Anne Dargassies, (1952) Etudes neurologigues sur le nouveau-né et le jeune nourisson. 207, Paris.

André-Thomas et al., (1954) Presse méd. 146 885

Arnheim, R., (1969) Visual thinking. University of California Press, Berkely, CA.

Ayres, A.J., (1979/82) Sensory integration and the child. Western Psychological Services, Los Angeles, CA.

Bainbridge Cohen, B., (1993) Sensing, feeling and action. Contact Editions, P.O. Box 603, Northampton, MA 01061

Bakker, D.J., (1990) Neurophysiological treatment of dyslexia. Oxford University Press Inc.

Bax M., Whitmore K., (1999) cited in Whitmore K, Hart H, Willems G (eds) A neurodevelopmental approach to specific learning disorders. Whitmore K, Hart H, Willems G., Mackeith, London.

Bein-Wierzbinski W., (2001) Persistent primitive reflexes in elementary school children. Effect on oculomotor and visual perception. Paper presented at the 13th European Conference of Neuro-Developmental Delay in Children with Specific Learning Difficulties. Chester, UK.

Bell, C, Magendie F., (1820) On the nerves of the orbit. Philosophical Transactions of the Royal Society 113 289-307

Bender, M.L., (1976) Bender-Purdue reflex test. Academic Therapy Publications. San Rafael, CA.

Benett, R., (1988) The hidden Moro. Private publication.

Bernhardsson, K., Davidson, K., (1982) *Ett Annorlundo sät att hjälpa med inlärningssvärigheter.* The Educational Psychology Department, Gothenburg Education Authority, Sweden.

Bernhardsson, K., Davidson, K., (1983) A different way of helping children with learning difficulties. A final report from the Dala Clinic (in Swedish). The Educational Psychology Department, Gothenburg Education Authority, Sweden.

Bertolotti, M., (1904) Rev. Neurol (Fr) 12 1160,202.42(1912)

Beuret, L., (2000) The role of postural reflexes in learning, pt. 2 Paper presented to the 12th Conference of Neuro-Developmental Delay in Children with Specific Learning Difficulties, Chester, UK.

Beuret, L. (1989) personal communication.

Bloedal, J.R., Brachfa V., (1997) Duality of cerebellar motor and cognitive function. International Review of Neurobiology. 41 Academic Press.

Blythe, P., (1971) Hypnotism, its power and practice. Arthur Barker, London.

Blythe, P. (1976) Self Hypnotism. Arthur Barker, London and Taplinger, NY.

Blythe, P., (1990) An organic basis for panic disorder and anxiety. Paper presented at the 4th International Conference of Neuro-Developmental Delay. Guernsey. C.I.

Blythe, P. (1990) A physical basis for panic disorder. Lecture at the 4th International Conference of Neurological Dysfunction in Children and Adults. Guernsey, C. UK, September, 1990.

Blythe, P. and McGlown, D.J., (1979) An organic basis for neuroses and educational difficulties. Insight Publications, 4 Stanley Place, Chester, UK.

Blythe, P., (1992) Personal communication.

Bobath, K. and Bobath B., (1955) Tonic reflexes and righting reflexes in the diagnosis and assessment of Cerebral Palsy. Cerebral Palsy Bulletin, May 16, 1955.

Bobath, B., (1975) Abnormal postural reflex activity caused by brain lesions. William Heineman, London.

Brain, W. B., (1987) Brain's clinical neurology. Revised by Bannister, R., Oxford Medical Publications, Oxford.

Brunnström, S., (1962) Training the adult hemiplegic patient: orientation of techniques to patients' motor behaviour. In: Approaches to treatment of patients with neuromotor dysfunction. 3rd International Congress, World Federation of Occupational Therapists.

Brunnström, S., (1970) *Movement therapy in hemiplegia: a neuro-physiological approach.* Harper and Row, New York.

Butler Hall B., (1998) Discovering the hidden treasures in the ear Paper presented at the 10th European Conference of Neuro-Developmental Delay in Children with Specific Learning Difficulties. Chester, UK.

Capute, A. (1986) Early neuro-motor reflexes in infancy. Pediatric Annals, March 15,1986.

Capute, A., Shapiro B.K. Palmer, F.B., Accardo, PJ. Wachtel, R.C., (1981) Primitive reflexes, a factor in non-verbal language in early infancy. Language Behaviour in Infancy and Early Childhood. (Ed. Stark.) Elsevier North Holland, Rue, Netherlands.

Cherqui, S., (2000) De, L'invie a L'acquis des reflexes primitives aux reflexes posturaux. Le traitement osteopathique comme facteur d'integration des functions cerebrales. Mémoire de Madame Mauriette, Sarah Cherqui. Pour la soutenance du diplome d'osteopathie. DO

Clements S.D., (1966) Task force one. Minimal brain dysfunction in children.

Cottrell, S., (1987) Aetiology, diagnosis and treatment of asthma through primitive reflex inhibition. Presented at the 2nd International Conference of Neurological dysfunction. Stockholm, 1988.

Courchesne, E. Townsend, J., Saitoh, O., (1994) The Brain in infantile autism. Posterior fossa structures are abnormal. Neurology 44 214-223

Cratty, B.J., (1973)Movemens, behavior and motor learning. Henry Kimpton Publishers, London.

Dalcroze, E.J. (1991) Cited in Dalcoze today - an education through and into music. Bachman, M.L. Clarendon Press, Oxford.

De Klein, Magnus R, (1924) Experimentell Physiologie des Vestibulapparatus. Handbuch der Neurologie des Ohresheilkunde. 1.

Delacato, C.H., (1959) The treatment and prevention of reading problems. Charles C. Thomas, Springfield, Illinois.

Delacato, C. H., (1974) The ultimate stranger, the autistic child. Academic Therapy Publications, Novato, CA.

DeMyer, W. (1980), Techniques of the neurological examination. McGraw-Hill, New York.

Dennison, P.E., (1981) Switching on. Edu-Kinesthetics, Glendale, CA.

Diamond S., Balvin R., Diamond R., (1963) Inhibition and choice. Harper Rowe, NY.

Dickson, V., Personal communication.

Draper, I.T., (1993) Lecture notes on neurology. Blackwell Scientific Publications, Oxford.

Duighan, (1994) personal communication.

Eustis, R.S., (1947) The primary origin of the specific language disability. Journal of Pediatrics XXXI (1947)

Faulkner, P., (1988) *The detection of neuro-physiological factors in children with reading problems.* Paper presented at the 2nd International Conference of Neurological Dysfunction. Stockholm, Sweden.

Faulkner, P., (1989) *The detection of neuro-physiological factors in children with reading problems.* Paper given at the Second International Conference on Children with Neuro-developmental Delay, Chester, UK.

Fay, T., (1958) Neuromuscular reflex therapy for spastic disorders. The Journal of the Florida Medical Association. 44 1234-1240

Fay, T., An overview of his life and works. Eds. Wolf J.D., Henderson A.R. A collection of undated, unpublished papers.

Fay, T., (1942) quoted in Doman G., Le Winn, E.B., Wilkinson, R., (1977) Temple Fay revisited: "The other side of the fit." A bill of particulars on seizures and on discontinuing anticonvulsant drugs. The In-Report. Vol V, no. 6, 1977.

Field, J., (1992) Accommodating the neuro-developmentally delayed child within the classroom. Field Publications, Gatepiece Cottage, Highfields, Wichenford, Worcester, UK.

Field, J. and Blythe, P., (1988) Towards developmental re-education. Field Publication, Gatepiece Cottage, Highfields, Wichenford, Worcester, UK.

Finger, S., (2000) Minds behind the brain. A history of the pioneers and their discoveries. Oxford University Press.

Fiorentino, M.R., (1981) Reflex testing methods for evaluating C.N.S. development. Bannerstone House, 301327 East Lawrence Ave., Springfield, Ill.

Flourens, M.J.P., (1924) Recherches éxperimentales sur les proriétés et les functions du systeme nerveux des animaux vertebras.

Frostig, M., (1970) Movement education: theory and practice. Follett Publishing Company, Chicago.

Gaddes, W.H., (1980) Learning disabilities and brain function: a neurophysical approach. Springer Verlag, New York.

Galaburda, A.M., LeMay, M., Kemper, T.L. Geschwind, N., (1978) Right/left asymmetries in the brain. Harvard University Press, Massachusetts.

Galaburda, A., (2001) Dyslexia and the brain. Paper presented at the 5th British Dyslexia Association International Conference. University of York. April 2001

Galant, S., (1917) Der Rückgratreflex. Diss. Basel

Galley, P.M. & Forster, A.L., (1982) Human movement. Churchill Livingston, Edingburgh.

Ganong, W.F., (1997) Review of medical physiology. Appleton and Lange. Stamford, Connecticut.

Gazzaniga, M.S., (1973) Brain theory and minimal brain dysfunction. Annals of the New York Academy of Sciences 205

Gesell, A., (1947) Part 1, The first five years of life. A guide to the study of pre-school children. Wathuen, 36 Essex Street, Strand. London.

Gesell, A. and Ames, L., (1947) The development of handedness, Journal of Genetic Psychology, 70 1941 pp 155-75.

Gilfoyle, E., Grady A. & Moore, J. (1972) Children adapt. Ch. Slack Inc. 6900 Grove Rd. Thorofare, N.J.

Goddard, S., (1989) The Fear paralysis response and its interaction with the primitive reflexes. INPP Monograph Series., No.1,1989, Chester, England.

Goddard, S., (1989) The fear paralysis reflex and its interactions with the primitive reflexes. Private publication.

Goddard Blythe, S., Hyland D., (1998) Screening for neurological dysfunction in the specific learning difficulty child. The British Journal of Occupational Therapy 10 1998

Goddard Blythe, S., (2001) Neurological Dysfunction as a significant factor in children diagnosed with dyslexia. Proceedings of The 5th International British Dyslexia Association Conference. University of York. April, 2001

Gold, S. J., (1998) If Kids Just Came with Instruction Sheets. Fern Ridge Press, Eugene, OR.

Gustafsson, D., (1970) A comparison of basic reflexes with the subtests of the Purdue perceptual-motor survey. Unpublished Master's Thesis. University of Kansas.

Guyton, A.C., (1991) Basic neuroscience - anatomy and physiology. W.B. Saunders Company, Philadelphia, PA.

Hagberg, B., (1975) Minimal brain dysfunction in children. Sätryck ur Läkartidningen 72 329-330

Hallett, M., Grafman J., (1996) Executive function and motor skill learning. Internatial Review of Neurobiology, 41 Academic Press

Hocking, B., (1990) Little boy lost. Bloomsbury Publishing Ltd, London.

Hobson, Allan P.,(1988) The dreaming brain. Basic Books,

Holt, K.S., (1991) Child Development. Butterworth-Heineman, London.

Hubbard, D.G., (1971) The skyjacker: his flights of fantasy. Collier Macmillan, New York and London.

Ingram, T.T.S., (1973) Soft signs. Dcv. Med. Child Neurol. 15 527

Ivry, R.B., Keele S.W., (1989) Timing functions of the cerebellum. Journal of Cognitive Neuroscience. 1 136-152.

Johansen, K.V., (1993) Lyd, Horelseog sprogudvikling. Dyslexia Research Lab. Ro Skolovej 14 DK 3760, Gudhjem, Bornholm, Denmark.

Johansen, K.V., (1992) Sensory deprivation-a possible cause of dyslexia. Nordisk Tidsskrift for Spesialpedagogikk, Scandinavian University Press Abonementssekjonen, Postboks 2959, Toyen, N-0608 Oslo, Norge.

Kaada, B., (1986) Sudden Infant Death Syndrome. Oslo University Press.

Kaada, B., (1988) Electrocardio response associated with the fear paralysis response in infant rabbits and rats. Presented at Rogaland Central Hospital, Jan. 1988. Functional Neurology 4(4) 1989

Kaada, B., Felman, R.S., Langfeldt, T., (1975) Failure to modulate autonomic reflex discharge by hippocampal stimulation in rabbits. Physiol. Behav. 7 225-231.

Kandel, Eric., Schwartz, J.H., Jessell, T.M., (1991) Principles of Neural Science, Third Edition. Appleton & Lange, Norwalk, Connecticut.

Kavale, K., Mattson, D.P., (1983) One jumped off the balance beam. Journal of Learning Disabilities 3/83.

Keeling, E., (2000) personal communication

Kephart, N.C., (1960) The slow learner in the classroom. Merrill, Columbus, Ohio.

Kermoian, Rosanne, (1988) Locomotor experience: A facilitator of spatial cognitive development. Child Development, Aug. 1988, Vol. 59.

King, L.J., Schrager O.L., (1999) A sensory and cognitive approach to the assessment and remediation of developmental learning and behavioral disorders. Paper presented at Symposium, Atlanta, Georgia.

Kiphard, E.J., (2000) Intervention program using the German psycho-motor approach with exceptional children. The 13th European Conference of Neuro-Developmental Delay in Children with Specific Learning Difficulties. Chester, UK.

Laborit, H., (1952) As quoted in Odent. M. Birth reborn.

Landsberg, P.G. (1975) Bradycardia during human diving. South African Medical Journal, 49 (15) 626-30

Larsell, (1947) The cerebellum of myxinoids and petromyzonts including developmental stages in the lampreys. Journal of Comp. Neurology, 86 395

Lefroy, R., (1990) Improving literacy through motor development. Dunsborough Enterprises. Pty Ltd Publications, P.O. Box 134, Palmyra, W. Australia 6157.

Leiner, H.C., Leiner, A.L., Dow, R.S., (1986) Does the cerebellum contribute to mental skills? Behav. Neuroscience. 100 443-454.

Leiner, H.C., Leiner, A.L., Dow, R.S., (1993) Cognitive and language functions of the human cerebellum. Trends in Neuroscience. 16.444-447

Le Mee, K. (1994) Chant. Random House, London.

Levinson, H.L., (1984) Smart but feeling dumb. Warner Books Inc., New York.

Levinson, H.L. (1986) Phobia Free. M. Evans & Co. Inc. New York.

Levinson, H.L. (1991) The upside down kids. M Evans & Co. Inc. New York.

Le Winn E.B., (1969) Human neurological organization. Charles C. Thomas, Illinois.

Lorente de No, R., (1933) Vestibular-ocular reflex. Archives of Neurology and Psychiatry. 30. 245-291

Machover, I. (1990) Personal communication.

MacLean, P., (1978) A mind of three minds: educating the triune brain. The National Society for the Study of Education, Chicago.

Madaule, P., (1993) When listening comes alive. Moulin Publishing, Box # 560, Ontario LOP IKO.

Martin, M., Grover B., (1990) Ears and hearing. Macdonald & Co. Ltd., Orbit House, London.

McPhillips, M., Hepper, P.G., Mulhern, G. (2000) Effects of replicating primary reflex movements on specific reading difficulties in children: a randomized, double-blind, controlled trial. The Lancet, Vol. 355, 2/2000.

Merck Manual, (1987) The manual of diagnosis and therapy (15th edition) Merck, Sharp & Dohme Research Laboratories.

Middlemiss, J., (1987) The Dalcroze project in East Herfordshire

Nicolson, R.I., Fawcett A.J., (1993) Early diagnosis of Dyslexia: An historic opportunity. Paper presented at the British Dyslexia Association "Early Diagnosis" Conference. Manchester. September 1993

Nicolson, R., Fawcett, A. Dean, P., (1994) Impaired performance of children with dyslexia on a range of cerebellar tests. Annals of Dyslexia. 46.259-283

Noica, (1912) Rev. Neurol. 20 I, 134

O'Dell N., Cook P., (1996) Stopping hyperactivity - a new solution. Avery Publishing Group, Garden City Park, New York.

Odent, M., (1991) Paper presented at The European Conference of Neuro-developmental Delay. Chester, UK.

Odent, M., (1986) Primal Health, Century, Hutchinson, London.

Odent, M., (1984) Birth reborn. Souvenir Press, London.

O'Reilly, B. (1990) The role of phenolic and related compounds as a possible causative factor in autism - a hypothesis. Private publication.

Pavlidis, 0., Miles, T., (1987) Dyslexia research and its applications to education. Wiley Publications.

Panskepp, J. (1998) Affective Neuroscience. Oxford University Press, Oxford.

Peiper A., (1963) Cerebral function in infancy and early childhood. The International Behavioral Sciences Series. New York.

Phillips, K., (1994) Contribution made to seminar. Chester, UK.

Portwood, M., (2001) Personal Communication to Peter Blythe.

Posner, M.I., Raichle, M.E., (1994) Images of mind. Freeman, New York.

Prochaska, G., (1784) Cited in: Neurobiology (1994) Shepherd GM., Oxford University Press.

Pulgar Marx, I. and P. De, (1955) Rev. Espan. Dedlat. 11317; see also Zentralb. Kinderheilk. 58 220, 1957.

Pyfer, J., Johnson R. (1981) Factors affecting motor delays. Extract from Adapted Physical Activity. Eason, Smith & Caron, Human Kinetics Publishers, Box 5076, Champaign, III. 618-20

Restak, R., (1991) The brain has a mind of its own. Harmony Books, New York.

Reuven, Kohen-Raz, (1986) Learning disabilities and postural control. Freund Publishing House Ltd. Suite 500, Chesham House, 150 Regent Street, London.

Rider, B., (1972) Relationship of postural reflexes to learning disabilities. American Journal of Occupational Therapy 26/5 239-243

Rowe, N. (1996) personal communication.

Schilder, P., (1933) The vestibular apparatus in neuroses and psychoses. Journal of Nervous and Mental Disease. 78 1-23, 137-164.

Schore, A.N., (1994) Affect regulation and the origin of the self. Laurence Erlbaum Associates. Hove, U.K.

Schrager, O.L., (1998) A sensory and cognitive approach to the assessment and remediation of developmental learning and behavioral disorders. Paper presented at Symposium, Atlanta, Georgia.

Schrager, 0.L., (2001) Posture and balance; important markers for children's learning development. Paper presented at the 13th Conference of Neuro-Developmental Delay in Children with Specific Learning Difficulties. Chester, UK.

Shaskan, D.A., Roller W.L., (1985) Paul Schilder. Mind explorer. Human Sciences Press. New York.

Shaywitz, S.E., (1996) Dyslexia. Scientific American, Nov. 77-83.

Shepherd, R., (1990) Physiotherapy in Pediatrics. Butterworth-Heineman, Oxford.

Sherrington, C., (1906) The integrative action of the nervous system. Yale University Press. New Haven, CT.

Smith, J., (1993) Illustrations. Flexton Bank, Tilston, Malpas, England.

Snider, R.S., Stowell, A., (1994) Receiving areas of the tactile, auditory and visual systems in the cerebellum. Journal of Neurophysiol. 7.331-357

Snowden, D., (2001) Ageing with Grace. Fourth Estate, London.

Southall, D.P., Samuels, M.P. & Talbert, D.G., (1990) Recurrent cyanotic episodes with severe arterial hypoxaemia and intrapulmonary shunting: a mechanism for sudden death. Archives of Disease in Childhood. 65:953-961

Steffert, B., (1997) Sign minds and design minds. Paper presented at the 9th European Conference of Nauro-Developmental Delay in Children with Specific Learning Difficulties. Chester, UK.

Steinbach, I., (1994) How does sound therapy work? Paper presented at The 6th European Conference of Neuro-Developmental Delay in Children with Specific Learning Difficulties. Klangstudio Lambdoma, Markgrafenufer 9,59071 Hamm, Germany.

Storr, A., (1993) Music and the mind. Harper Collins, 77-85 Fulham Palace Road, London.

Strauss, H., (1929) Journal of Psychology 38 111

Tallal, P, Piercy, M. (1974) Developmental aphasia: rate of auditory processing and selective impairment of consonantal perception. Neuropsychologia 12 83-98

Tansley, A.E., (1967) Reading and remedial reading. Routledge and Kegan Paul Ltd. London.

Telleus, C., (1980) En komarativ studie av neurologisk skillnader hos born medoch utan lsoch skrivovarigheter. Gotheborg Universitet, Psychologisker Instituktionen.

Thelan, F., (1979), Rhythmical stereotypes in normal human infants. Animal Behavior, 1979, 27 699-715

Ten Hoopen, J., (1995) personal communication.

Tomatis, A.A., (1991) The conscious ear. Station Hill Press Inc. Tarrytown, New York.

Tomatis, A.A. (1991) About the Tomatis method. The Listening Centre. 600 Markham Street, Toronto, Ontario, M6G 2LG.

Tomatis, A.A., (1980) Audio-psycho-phonology: a new challenge. Lecture given at Potchefstrom University, Republic of South Africa, April, 1980.

Trevor-Roper, P., (1987) The world through blunted vision. Penguin, London.

Veragruth, (1917) Neurol. Zbl., 1918, No.7

Veras, R., (1975) Children of dreams, children of hope. Henry Regnery, Chicago.

Wender, P.H., (1971) Minimal brain dysfunction in children. Whiley International, New York.

Whytt, R., (1751) An essay on the vital and other involuntary motions of the animaL Hamilton, Balfour and Neil. Edinburgh.

Wilkinson, G., (1994) The relationship of primitive postural reflexes to learning difficulty and underachievement ~ Unpublished M.Ed thesis. University of Newcastle-upon-Tyne.

Williamson, (1992) The Brain: science opens new windows on the mind. Newsweek, April 1992.

Willis T., (1670) On muscular movement

Wisbey, A., (1977) Sounding out dyslexia. World Medicine, London. October 1977.

Appendix 6

INDEX

Reticular activating system 43,
45, 154 ff
Reticular formation 43, 145, 154
Right brain, left brain functions
49 ff, 72, 103, 114, 134, 148, 152
Righting reflexes 31ff
Ritalin 137, 158
Roooting reflex 13 ff, 60
Rote learning 45, 105
Saccades 146
Salivary gland secretion 56
Schizophrenia 141
School readiness, xvi, 97 ff
Scoliosis 17
Segmental rolling reflex 35
Seizures 154
Selective mutism 141 ff
Self-esteem 7
Self-stimulation 63
Semicircular canals 57
Sensation 43ff, 79
Sense of direction 18
Sense of time 20
Sensory deprivation 57
Sensory integration 19, 39, 41
73, 101, 112
Sensory integration, A.J. Ayers 36
Sequential learning 39
Sequencing skills 20, 21, 37, 114
Sexual awareness 63, 78
Short attention span 55
see also hyperactivity
Short-term memory 17
Shyness 103,141ff
Smell 77 ff
Social problems 28, 33, 37, 44,
98 ff, 122, 133, 137, 141ff
Somatosensory map 60
Sound therapy 108ff
Space perception 19, 21, 103
Speech 8,9, 13, 14, 69, 126, 134,
141ff, 147, 157
Spelling 12, 50, 70, 72, 111,
113, 160
Spinal Galant xiii, 15 ff, 113
Splinter skill 77
Sports 11, 17, 20, 35, 63, 76
Stapedius muscle 38, 64
Startle Response, 8, 28, 30,
38, 151
Stimulus Bound effect 7, 12
Strauss (startle reflex) 5, 26,
36, 151
Sucking 8
Sudden Infant Death syndrome
10, 28 ff, 147, 148, 154, 158
Swallowing 14, 134
Swimming 20, 25, 127
Symmetrical Tonic Neck Reflex
19, 21 ff, 100, 113, 125

Sympathetic Nervous System 56
see also Fight or Flight
Tactility 4, 60 ff
Discriminative receptors 60
Hypotactility 60
Protective receptors 61
Tactile defensive 63
Tansley Standard Figures 72, 75
Taste 77 ff
Teaching strategies, 2, 97 ff
Temper tantrums 139, 146
Temperature controls 63, 149
Thalamus 43 ff
Theory of replication 100
Thumb opposition 9
Ticklishness 88, 155
Tonic Labyrinthine reflex 17, 22,
73, 99, 100, 150 ff,
Touch, 60ff
Triune brain 51
Unilaterality in brain function
51, 66, 149
see also dominance
Urination 16
Vagus nerve 145 , 157
Vallergan 158
Vestibular-ocular reflex arc
19, 58, 59, 73
Vestibulo-ocular motor skills
19, 34
Vestibular system 19, 56ff, 72,
102, 105, 133, 135, 145, 150,
153, 158
Vestibular stimulation 9, 105 ff,
159
Vision 12, 20 ff, 55, 59, 70 ff,
105, 111
Accomodation 71
Convergence 71, 72
Focus 23. 71
Myopia 72
Ocular pursuit 12
Pupillary reflex 7
Tracking 12, 72, 111
Visual-perceptual 7, 70, 73, 120
Visual-motor integration 11, 22,
111, 121, 125 ff, 133
Visual fixation 11, 23
Vocalization 107
Walking 11, 17, 25, 34, 59, 126,
159
Weight gain 61
Withdrawal 45, 60, 141 ff,
147, 153
Withdrawal reflexes 3, 4, 28, 156
Writing 24, 37, 50ff, 113, 125ff,
134, 136, 160
Xinguana Indians 24

NAMES INDEX

Alvegård, C. J., xi, 71, 131
Ames, Louise B., xvi, 51, 146
André-Thomas, S. A. D., 9
Arnheim, R., 6
Ayres, A.J., 18, 36, 41, 60, 101,
124, 148
Bakker, D.J., 50
Bax and Whitmore, xvi
Bein-Wierzbinski., W., 24, 128
Bell, C., 119
Bender, M, 24, 125
Bennett, R, 30, 83, 151
Berard, G., 16, 106
Bernhardsson, K., 127
Bertolotti, M., 15
Beuret, L., xi, 16, 37, 133, 137ff,
Bloedel, 28, 45
Blythe, P., xi, 23, 121, 122, 126
131, 135, 145, 147, 148, 157
Bobath, B., 22
Bobath, K., 22, 123, 146
Brachfa, V., 28, 45
Brain, W.B., 154
Brunnström, S., 147
Butler Hall, B., 16
Carlsson, H., xi
Caput, A., 22, 143, 150, 152
Changeux, J.P., xiii
Cherqui, S., 129
Clarke, S., 83
Clements, S.D., 122
Cook, P., 24, 25, 126
Cottrell, S., 152
Courchesne, E., 133
Cratty, B.J., 101, 124
Dalcroze, E. J., 109
Davidson, K., 127
Dale, H.H., 120
DeKlein, 135
Delacato, C.H., 41, 55, 121, 124
DeMyer, W., 10
Dennison, P.E., 101
Diamond, M., 136
Dickson, V. 16
Dobie, S., xi, 114
Doman, G., 41, 124
Dow, R.S., 104, 133
Draper, I.T., 133
Duighan, 72
Eustis, R.S., 149
Faulkner, J., 128
Fawcett, xvii , 134
Fay, T., 124, 154
Field, J., 112
Finger, S., 119
Fiorentino, M. R., 53
Flourens, M.J.P., 133
Frostig, M.124

*For test demonstrations and interview with
Peter Blythe and Sally Goddard, the following
VHS video is available . . .*

*For video in the **PAL** format
remit $30.00 U.S. (or equivalent foreign currency) plus
additional $5.00 U.S. for overseas postage.*

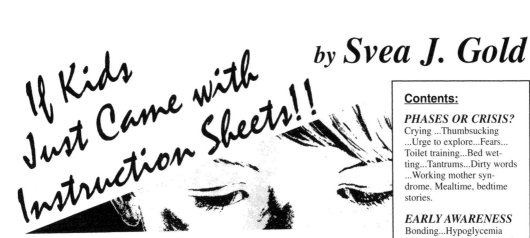

If Kids Just Came with Instruction Sheets!!

by Svea J. Gold

Contents:

PHASES OR CRISIS?
Crying ...Thumbsucking ...Urge to explore...Fears... Toilet training...Bed wetting...Tantrums...Dirty words ...Working mother syndrome. Mealtime, bedtime stories.

EARLY AWARENESS
Bonding...Hypoglycemia ...Allergies...Developmental problems...Sensitivity differences. **Debunking labels that paralyze: ADD, MBD, Dyslexia, Autism, Behavior problems.**

TEEN CHALLENGES
Normal separation or delinquency? Hormonal changes ... Nutrition needs ... Genetic tendencies. Behind delinquency: Drug abuse ... Prior sexual abuse ... Trauma ... Learning problems.

APPENDIX:
Stimulating a baby ... Testing for allergies...Evaluating and normalizing sensory distortions ... Brain development. **Program with delinquents: A new approach, not what comes out of a child, but what does not go in or not connect.** Quick functional neurological evaluation...Developmental techniques used and rationale for each procedure.

. . . and MORE!

Babies do not come in carefully dehydrated, precooked packages to which you simply add milk and love and who then will automatically grow into competent adults.

Your two-year-old will most likely run gleefully out the front door —naked as the day he was born! The four-year-old will call you dirty names and the teen will carefully ignore all parental advice!

When the little darlings start acting like children and not like the perfect angels of our fantasies, it is time to do some detective work. Is the child going through a phase or is there an underlying problem?

But a problem is not a problem if you can fix it —whether we are raising our own children or helping those of the global village. This book deals with connections, not just single answers. Whether we are exploring behavior problems, delinquency or drug abuse, rarely does just one remedy apply. Neither do all remedies apply to every child!

Even if only one of the many approaches suggested here helps only one child in a hundred, and that one child in a hundred is your child or a child in your acquaintance, this may be the most important book you ever read.